Praise for
Crusade against Cancers:
The Quest for Truth

"Your book is an eye-opener and is emotionally charged!

I believe all my students at New Eden School need to read this book so they can see what people go through in this battle against cancer, the patient and the family members. It's an excellent resource for tomorrow's natural health professionals.

God bless you for your efforts of love for Jerry, and really, for all of us!"

—Lawrence DeSantis, CFMP, ND
Director,
New Eden School of Natural Health and Herbal Studies

"Just finished the book and I couldn't wait to tell you . . . you have done an amazing job. We would like to keep a copy at our clinic and recommend this book to cancer patients as well as their families.

I am sure you will help many to think about taking control of their health."

—Kathy Jenkins
Manager and certified naturopath,
Budwig Center, a Natural Integrative Treatment Cancer Clinic,
Málaga, Spain

"Diane has done a masterful job helping the reader to understand cancer and the repercussions of traditional treatment. This compelling story makes you want to know more and delve into the resources for greater detail.

Crusade Against Cancers has the ability to change the tide in how we look at cancer treatment and the health cost to our families and environment."

—Jim Mullowney
Founder and CEO,
Pharma-Cycle

Crusade against Cancers:
The Quest for Truth

by Diane Bishop Hussey
with Jerry W. Hussey

Crusade against Cancers: The Quest for Truth
Published by Revelation Boulevard Publishing
PO Box 584
Wonder Lake, Illinois 60097
United States of America

ISBN 13: 978-1-7344994-0-7

Author photographs by Jared Silver, Executive Portrait Specialists
Cover design by Jim Saurbaugh, JS Graphic Design

Scripture quotations marked CSB have been taken from the Christian Standard Bible®, Copyright © 2017 by Holman Bible Publishers. Used by permission. Christian Standard Bible•, and CSB® are federally registered trademarks of Holman Bible Publishers.

Scripture quotations marked ESV are from The ESV® Bible (The Holy Bible, English Standard Version®), copyright © 2001 by Crossway, a publishing ministry of Good News Publishers. Used by permission. All rights reserved.

Scripture marked NCV taken from the New Century Version®. Copyright © 2005 by Thomas Nelson. Used by permission. All rights reserved.

Scripture quotations marked NIV are taken from the Holy Bible, New International Version®, NIV®. Copyright © 1973, 1978, 1984, 2011 by Biblica, Inc.™ Used by permission of Zondervan. All rights reserved worldwide.

DISCLAIMER: I, the author, am *NOT* a doctor or scientist, and I write from my personal education, extensive research, experience, and wisdom, wisdom acquired through the Bible and revelation from my Lord and Savior. None of the statements in this book has been evaluated by the FDA. This book does not claim, nor is it intended, to diagnose, treat, cure, or prevent any type of disease. The information provided is intended for your general knowledge only and is not a substitute for a physician's medical advice or treatment for any specific medical condition. Always seek the advice of your doctor or other qualified health care professional and institution with anything regarding a medical condition. Never disregard medical advice or delay in seeking it because of something you read in this book. My goal in writing is that you move forward with more complete information, not dismiss or ignore any information.

www.DianeBishopHussey.com
www.RevelationBoulevardPublishing.com

This book is dedicated to all who have cancer,
who have had cancer,
or will have cancer,
their families, friends, and loved ones.

I pray that this book not only empowers and equips
but also gives you hope and peace.

Contents

Part 1
The Oncology Experience

Part 2
The Natural Health Experience

Part 3
Cancer Today

Part 1
The Oncology Experience

Chapter 1
The Journey Begins

CANCER. The word alone evokes a strong response. It stirs up emotions, none of them positive. Some people visibly shudder at the word like they've had a sentence pronounced over them. Many get angry, depressed, nauseous, anxious, or numb. Others have so much fear that they can't even utter the word. Instead they refer to it as *the "C" word.*

How does someone's cancer journey begin? Often cancer is the furthest thing from their mind. They may go to the doctor for a minor ailment without any major symptoms, perhaps just a nagging pain, cough, or digestive issues. Routine testing may yield questionable findings that require additional tests. Other times people have a suspicion or fear about a lump or mole.

Some may run to the doctor to have their symptoms checked out, while others slip into denial and avoid going to the doctor for as long as possible.

When cancer is diagnosed, more testing is done to home in on treatment. Decisions have to be made, and there are a multitude of variables. Where is the cancer located? What stage is it? Is it contained, or has it spread? What is the person's age, and how healthy or strong are they? Do they have insurance, and what does it cover?

A cancer diagnosis comes with countless unknowns. It's overwhelming on so many levels. And often most unnerving is that the word itself can feel like one's fate has been pronounced.

However, cancer doesn't have to be a sentence. Not at all. There are other options, methods of holistic, alternative approaches, with high rates of not only survival, but also total and lasting recovery from cancer. This is what my husband, Jerry, and I learned firsthand.

Simply put, there are many key factors to achieving victory, but to me four stand out as particularly important.

First, choose life, because healing from cancer *is* a choice. When Jerry no longer had any options available through the medical system, we turned to alternative health. So, I can speak to both the conventional medical treatment he received and the natural health options we experienced. Understanding both approaches is critical.

At the point Jerry opted for alternative health, we chose life, totally engaging in life through natural, holistic healing. We did our research, made changes, and believed in the proven science. And as Jerry became actively involved in his own health care decisions, his resolve to not only choose life but to *live* it increased dramatically.

Second, choose your attitude, and make it a good one. That's what Jerry and I did, and that's why we had an amazing story. Choosing and keeping a positive mental attitude brings hope. A positive attitude has been shown to greatly improve psychological and physical well-being. I've heard that doctors can predict with 80 percent accuracy who is going to make it, based solely on their attitude.

Third, choose to be equipped. We need the knowledge, training, and tools to make well-informed decisions. Let's create a brief scenario to give perspective. In our analogy, an average person, with no medical background, is diagnosed with cancer. Typically they have done little, if any, research. Since cancer is often referred to as a battle, our personal war against a horrendous disease, let's view cancer as a military battle.

Imagine that this average individual has been drafted, and there just isn't time for boot camp to get him prepared. He's told it's essential he go into battle immediately. The leader says, "Trust me, and just do what I tell you. Simply follow my directions."

The draftee has no equipment, no training, and no idea what to expect. Does his going into battle sound like a good plan? And yet that is what often happens when someone is diagnosed with cancer. The leader is the oncologist, and the patient is told what the treatment is and where to go for all the tests and procedures.

So what happens if your leader doesn't have adequate training, or doesn't have the most up-to-date, or most effective, information himself? After all, cancer still thrives today, despite the specialized field of oncology.

I like to think of this book not only as boot camp, providing a lot of the basics needed, but as tech school as well, to take you to the next level, so that you understand many effective options that are available.

Fourth, choose God. Although some may be put off by the mere mention of God, He has been a fundamental part of Jerry and my journey. As the trials from cancer increased, our reliance on God increased as well. We grew from a distant belief in God's existence to complete faith and trust in Him as a key part of our lives.

In short, I don't know how we would have made it without Him. It still touches me deeply every time I ponder how incredibly often God showed up and was actively involved in the details of our lives, even though Jerry and I hadn't been faith-filled people through most of our marriage. Although it's wonderful to be supported by family and friends, God multiplies the comfort, peace, strength, and healing exponentially.

Of those four, mostly this book is about hope, truth, and choosing life. As you read you will find science that reveals solutions for cancer already exist and have been saving lives around the world for more than seventy years.

My mind usually goes to the practical rather than the emotional, but my heart aches each time I learn that someone is diagnosed with cancer, because I have a good idea of the journey ahead of them. Jerry was diagnosed with cancer not once, or twice, but five times. For the first three cancers and part of his fourth, we did what the oncologists told us, like well-trained dogs. Jerry received chemotherapy, radiation, and surgery. Yet he kept getting new cancers, and his health increasingly suffered from side effects of the treatments.

During Jerry's fourth and fifth cancers, which he had simultaneously, we kept our family and friends updated on frequent developments through blogging on the CaringBridge website (www.CaringBridge.org). When we started the blog, Jerry said, "I want to keep everything positive. Let's not write anything that will cause our family to worry. We'll put off posting until we can put a positive spin on it." While journaling online, we remained true to our original intent—to leave our readers with a positive mindset. In the process, Jerry and I found ourselves renewed and uplifted, and so our attitude and story were nearly the complete opposite of the typical cancer scenario.

As our cancer story unfolded, many of our readers encouraged us, and then directly asked us, to turn our blogged story into a book. They said Jerry's cancer journey was encouraging, inspiring, and needed to be shared. There did seem to be a lot of interest in knowing more, but I felt ill-equipped to bring a book to fruition and set that notion aside.

As the years passed, I would tell people about Jerry's/our cancer journey, sharing the knowledge and experience we gained while living through two entirely different approaches to dealing with cancer. I found a deep desire to try to help people understand cancer and investigate natural health alternatives.

Finally, I started the book five years from the exact day Jerry went into the hospital the last time. Originally this book was intended to be fairly simple and straightforward, just copying and pasting blog posts from the CaringBridge website to show people how Jerry and I "did" his fourth and fifth cancers a different way. I added the basics—that Jerry was diagnosed with five cancers total over eleven years and how we went from chemo, radiation, and surgery to natural health.

I had to ponder and reflect as I attempted to write about Jerry's first three cancers. It was hard for me to remember because I always try to forget the negative, and generally I'm very good at it. Big events came to mind, but the details and emotions were hard to recall.

Because most of the manuscript was copied from Jerry's CaringBridge page, the rough draft basically wrote itself in just ten days. But it needed some help. I couldn't figure out how to start or end that version of the manuscript. So, I went to an editor for help.

She read through it. Afterward we sat down together, and I told her all the straightforward facts of Jerry and my cancer experiences. And then she gently asked one question: "Diane, what was your emotional journey?"

To be honest, I drew a blank. I'd kept my emotions walled up for years. But as she patiently questioned me and drew me out that day and over the months that followed, the wall came tumbling down. I thought it would hurt too much to go through it again, and I didn't want to hurt. The wall had kept me protected . . . and had kept me a prisoner.

During that time, she also asked me to provide dates of events for clarity. For that I pulled out Jerry's medical records, thinking I'd find quick, easy answers.

I'd had no idea it would start me down a path that would not only hijack the book from the original story line, but also take me into two of the most difficult, heart-wrenching years of my life.

While sifting through the stacks of medical records to look for dates, I discovered reports and doctors' notes with information so shocking I could hardly breathe. I found negligence, and even gross negligence bordering on medical malpractice.

It sent me, and this book, in a whole new direction. As I researched, I became angry and depressed as I uncovered lies, deceit, and outrageous statements in Jerry's medical records. The stack of records is more than five inches thick. I went through it half a dozen times or more, unable to let go until I'd found peace—until I felt certain all the clues had been unearthed, as well as the complete and honest truth.

Family and friends started to question why I continued to put myself through it. I'd hear, "You were so much happier before you started writing. Maybe you should just let it go."

But the pressure to write it continued to build to the point I simply had to. In my heart, I knew our journey would bless others. Sometimes people need wisdom and knowledge from someone who has gone before them.

If I didn't share what I knew, many people wouldn't have the opportunity to hear of a different, better way to battle and/or avoid cancer entirely. I needed to share our journey, Jerry's and mine, and all that we'd discovered along the way.

But I know that in our society, the odds are that people will go running to the oncologist just as Jerry and I did, like well-trained dogs. I know that analogy is hard to read, but that's how convicted and passionate I've become since I've discovered that there are solutions—solutions that modern medicine doesn't want the public to become aware of.

I still wanted the book to end on a positive and uplifting note. I wasn't sure how to do it. But I believe in the book and our story—a beautiful story, orchestrated by God from the very beginning. So, I'll trust God to lead the way.

My heart's desire is that it will create a hunger, passion, and urgency within you to join the growing crusade, that you start your own quest for truth. I pray it will lead you to a place where you are strengthened and equipped to fight the good fight yourself or in support of others. Most of all, I stand in faith that, with the proper equipment and training, we *will* win the battle over this disease.

Yes, the word *cancer* can be scary to hear, but I pray and trust that by the end of this book, you'll never fear the word or the diagnosis again.

On that note, permit me to share with you our story.

☐

Jerry's cancer journey began in early September 2000. We were blessed, living a fairly comfortable life in San Antonio, Texas. Our sons, Brandon and Devin, both pursuing careers, had moved out on their own. Tara, our youngest, attended college on a soccer scholarship. Jerry worked out of our home as a regional sales manager for a medical and industrial vacuum equipment company and traveled often. I enjoyed my job as branch manager for a lighting maintenance company.

It started simply enough. Jerry and a friend were fooling around, and the friend playfully hit him in the stomach. He wasn't hit hard, but a couple of days later his stomach still hurt.

Typically, men don't go to the doctor often, and Jerry was no exception. He hadn't been to the doctor since long before we'd moved to Texas more than five years before. We felt a bit concerned, because in addition to the pain in his stomach, Jerry had been losing weight. With a little friendly encouragement from me, he finally decided to go to the family doctor. I'll call him "Dr. GP" (general practitioner).

Dr. GP asked numerous questions and did all the things doctors do. When Dr. GP felt Jerry's abdomen, he found an unmistakable mass. The doctor ordered a battery of tests.

First, Jerry went in for an ultrasound of his abdominal mass. A few days later, he had a CT scan (often referred to as a CAT scan) of his abdomen.

The abdominal ultrasound and CT scan showed that the mass in his abdomen was about the size of a large cantaloupe.

More tests would be needed to determine the cause of the mass, Dr. GP said, and he referred us to an oncologist. He stressed the importance of making that appointment as soon as possible after the testing was completed. The following week Jerry had three more tests: a biopsy of the abdominal mass, an ultrasound of the boys, and a CT of the chest.

Quite honestly, I think we were in a state of shock. We put one foot in front of the other, waiting for the oncologist appointment and the test results. Jerry and I weren't prone to worry, but oncologist means, at the very least, suspicion of cancer. We hoped that assumption was wrong, but I think both of us knew.

We were scheduled to meet with the oncologist on Friday.

Jerry and I steeled ourselves as we drove to the oncologist appointment. Neither of us said much. Instead we focused on being strong for each other. He and I had always been optimistic, so it wasn't our nature to give in to fear. We'd hear the test results and, if it was cancer, then the course of action.

The two of us made a good team. Earlier in the month, we'd celebrated our twenty-ninth wedding anniversary. Jerry and I weren't a couple who fought. Somehow, we knew what to say and what not to say. What one couldn't figure out, the other could. We complemented each other as we journeyed through life together. We had comfortable give and take, like the rhythm of the ocean, and together we relished our buoyant sense of humor.

We truly did have a blessed life, but we weren't strangers to hard times, which only served to make us stronger as individuals and as a team. It was that strength, love, and optimism that we drew upon during difficult times.

Even so, at the oncologist's office, nervousness crept in as we waited in the reception area. Thankfully, we only had a brief wait until we were shown into the doctor's office and sat down.

The oncologist pushed up his glasses and glanced across his desk at us. The open file of test results and notes lay between us. He briskly paged through the paperwork, refreshing his memory of the findings.

That done, he sat back, skipped any small talk or indication of personality, and bluntly led with the facts. "I have bad news, and I have good news. The bad news is that it's confirmed. The ultrasound revealed a dime-sized mass in the right testicle. Jerry does have testicular cancer, and it has spread to Jerry's abdomen."

In the short pause, I'm sure we tried to process what we'd just heard. We weren't people who tended to panic. Rather, we typically rolled along with life's ups and downs.

The oncologist went on. "That kind of cancer is more common in young men between the ages of fifteen and thirty-five. It's unusual for a man who's fifty-one, like Jerry. The good news is that testicular cancer has the best success rate of any cancer that a man can get, 95 percent. Those are good odds."

I looked over at Jerry and took hold of his hand. Those were good odds.

"The treatment plan consists of chemotherapy. That will kill the cancer. Due to the size of the mass in his abdomen, our first goal is to shrink that tumor. However, I have a concern for Jerry's kidneys, so Jerry will have to be admitted to the hospital for his first round of chemo."

Admitted to the hospital?

"Okay-y-y," Jerry said.

The oncologist wrote a few notes in the file. "The chemotherapy we'd normally use for testicular cancer is filtered by the kidneys, so we'll have to use a different chemo that will be filtered by the liver."

Neither Jerry nor I questioned the medical side of things further. His explanation didn't make sense to us, but he was the oncologist. We'd follow his advice.

He called to the nurse and asked her to check whether Jerry could be admitted to the hospital on Monday morning to start chemo.

With that detail being handled, he turned back to us. "Do you have any questions?"

My mind was swirling. I'm sure I had a million questions, but for the moment, I could only ask one. "Since Jerry has been diagnosed with cancer, should he give up smoking cigarettes?" I thought, *Undoubtedly the doctor will say that he should, and Jerry will give up the two-and-a-half packs a day habit.*

He pushed up his glasses again. "No, giving it up would be too stressful." He made another note.

WHAT? I couldn't conceive of someone with cancer smoking, no matter what type of cancer. It's just . . . unhealthy! The oncologist's response seemed so contrary to everything I'd heard. My mind felt boggled, and I couldn't think.

The silence grew deafening as Jerry and I sat there trying to deal with all we'd just heard. The nurse returned to advise the doctor that Jerry could, indeed, be admitted to the hospital Monday morning to start chemotherapy.

In retrospect, why didn't we look for another doctor, based on the doctor's thumbs-up to keep smoking? But I already knew the answer: Jerry wouldn't want to. He enjoyed smoking and had no desire to quit. The doctor had let him do just what he wanted.

I was beside myself. (I've made up names for all the oncologists we went to through the years, sometimes with a touch of cynicism. I began to think of this one as Dr. Blinders.) I took a deep breath, buried my frustration over the doctor's response, and compelled my mind to return to the conversation at hand. All of this was happening to Jerry—my Jerry—but he had a 95 percent chance of success.

Driving home, Jerry and I knew we were moving into uncharted territory. Neither of us had any close friends or relatives who had gone through cancer, and the Internet at the time wasn't what it is today. We certainly didn't know what we didn't know. So, we entrusted Jerry's health to the doctors and the medical system.

□

Three days later, the hospital admitted Jerry for a five-day stay while they gave him chemo and worked to stabilize his health. Of course, they put Jerry on the floor with the rest of the cancer patients, but we really didn't belong there because it's a very somber place.

Our whole family tends to deal with stressful situations with an abundance of humor. We were probably a bit loud and rambunctious, and that didn't work too well for Jerry's roommate. He was a cranky, elderly man who no longer understood the concept of modesty. He often lay with his covers thrown off and his hospital gown raised up. The man was buck-naked underneath. The staff, cognizant of our daughter Tara's age, respectfully moved Jerry to a private room to better accommodate his roommate's need for rest, and our desire for basic discretion.

Tara bought Jerry a reddish-purple betta fish to keep him company. Bowing to our comedic tendencies, she named the fish Chemo. Many businesses install aquariums to create an atmosphere of peace for their visitors, and Chemo offered that to us all.

Jerry endured three chemo cocktails over the first three days, with two types of chemo, carboplatin and VP-16®, in each. The bodily wastes were so toxic that he was told to flush the toilet twice every time he went.

He had the expected side effects of nausea, vomiting, and diarrhea, as well as fatigue, pain, and chills. One of the less common side effects Jerry experienced was a metallic taste during the infusion of the chemo VP-16. Not only did Jerry endure that unpleasant reaction, but it would also haunt him for years to come. Even if the metallic taste wasn't a side effect of chemotherapies that he would receive with subsequent cancer diagnoses, Jerry would still get that VP-16 taste. The experience had such an indelible impact on Jerry that he even had that metallic taste rise up one afternoon while driving, when he heard someone on the radio talking about her ordeal with cancer and chemotherapy.

As I recount the list of side effects of chemotherapy that Jerry experienced, I realize how clinical it sounds. Where are the emotions and details? As I've struggled to recall all that transpired, those memories are limited. In my opinion, they are best forgotten, if you're able. I don't think we are well served recalling the worst of times.

Jerry and I moved along, putting one foot in front of the other. Both of us kept up our natural optimism. Besides, Jerry had the most curable form of cancer a man can get, and we believed we had a good doctor. So, we believed he would be cured.

During those five days, Tara and I often walked through the halls alongside Jerry in his hospital garb. He pushed his IV pole with its bag as we headed to or from the elevator, so he could go to the roof and smoke.

After work, our sons, Brandon and Devin, came to visit. I can still see them strolling through the halls and smoking on the roof with their dad. Try as I may, I still cannot fathom why Jerry and the boys chose to smoke, especially since Jerry's father had died of emphysema years before I met Jerry.

☐

While Jerry was in the hospital, I received an unexpected call from the Blood and Tissue Center, requesting that I donate platelets for a child with leukemia. This young person happened to be in the same hospital as Jerry, albeit in the Children's Center.

I'd been a regular blood and platelet donor, until a nurse told me I shouldn't donate anymore because of the difficulty they had tapping into my veins. The center called since all my markers were a good match for a specific child who wasn't responding to the platelet donations he or she had been given. I thought platelet donations were generic but was told that a really good match might jumpstart their system and make a difference. They likened it to some people not responding to generic drugs, but who get results from the original medication.

I did donate and prayed that it was just what the child needed.

The only reason I included this tidbit is because we hear that what goes around comes around. Often we think of that saying negatively. But, as you will learn later in the story, Jerry was going to need platelets, and a lot of them.

Pay it forward when you are able, because you never know what you or a loved one might need in the future.

☐

The day Jerry was discharged, his doctor encouraged him to eat whatever he wanted, even big bowls of ice cream before bed, to regain some weight. He had lost more than forty pounds. He was also told to drink two quarts of Gatorade every day to balance the electrolytes.

When we returned home, Jerry dutifully followed the doctor's advice. I bought shopping carts stacked with frosty ice cream cartons and gallons of Gatorade, and we moved into the next phase of Jerry's chemotherapy.

Chapter 2
More Side Effects . . . and Difficult News

After Jerry was released from the hospital following his initial round of chemo, he reexperienced the bad flu-like side effects every three weeks—roughly one week awful, two weeks better—for a total of nine rounds of chemo over six and a half months. Always he flushed the toilet twice each time he went.

He also developed mouth sores, one of the worst side effects Jerry experienced. The mouth sores made it difficult to eat and drink for the duration of his chemotherapy and for weeks afterward. It hurt him to chew, and any foods or beverages that were even slightly acidic, salty, or spicy burned every sore in his mouth. Many times Jerry didn't want to eat or drink anything at all. Of course, that wasn't good, because the doctor wanted Jerry to regain some weight.

From his first day in the hospital, the medical team warned him how devastating chemo could be to his immune system. Basically, as chemo kills the cancer cells, it also destroys healthy cells and the immune system. Our white blood cell count (WBC) is an indication of our ability to fight infection. Ordinarily, chemotherapy causes the WBC count to drop drastically, which is why people receiving chemo often wear masks when they go out. Jerry, an exceptional patient, dutifully followed all the doctor's orders. He limited his participation in outside activities and contact with people.

Since Jerry worked out of our San Antonio home, he could fulfill his regular employment requirements by phone and e-mail. He had established and trained a network of distributors, so he was able to successfully manage his territory during the cancer treatments. He made few sales calls in person and took only a couple of brief sales trips.

Tara, in college, thrived in the midst of soccer season. Jerry loved watching Tara play, so he'd load a chair into the car, go to the soccer games with me, and sit far away from everyone. He took his mask with him but preferred to isolate rather than donning the mask.

People in cancer treatment may or may not lose their hair, depending on the type of chemotherapy used. Hair loss can be mentally and emotionally traumatic. Even at age fifty-one, Jerry had a nice, thick head of hair. Like so many other cancer patients, he was distressed by his hair falling out. He'd wake up in the morning and find clumps on his pillow. As he'd wash his hair, more and more accumulated in his hands and clogged the shower drain.

One morning he looked in the mirror and saw bald patches. Finally, reality set in. Disheartened, he said, "Diane, I can't stand it. Shave it off. All of it." And then, the wry grin. "At least Michael Jordan has made bald look cool."

It was a warm, sunny afternoon in late October when Jerry sat down outside at our patio table. He had no idea, since we chatted away and I kept him distracted, that I was giving him a "special" haircut before shaving his head completely. Ever the comedienne, I gave him a Mohawk.

Then I made some excuse, ran into the house, and grabbed the camera. The picture I took made him laugh, his hearty belly laugh. Afterward I shaved off the rest of his hair. Our kids wished we'd waited to shave his head so they could have seen the Mohawk, but we enjoyed a lot of laughs at the picture. We usually tried to find the good in not-so-good situations, or at least find the humor.

I don't think either of us ever got used to his new, bald look. He often wore hats, and we don't have any photographs of him without hair. Some people look good without hair, but mostly I think it's because they're healthy. When chemo causes people to lose their hair, they usually look sick since they've lost a lot of weight, tend to be fatigued, and just don't feel well. Jerry joked about his bald look, his scalp getting cold, and about being careful not to get sunburned. I loved him and his spirit even more.

Because he was easily fatigued and often felt ill, Jerry spent a lot of time on the computer. He started researching his family's ancestry online. It gave him something to do and focus on, distracting himself from the effects of the chemo. Fascinated, he traced back generation after generation, eventually tracing all the way to Hubert Hussey of Normandy, France, born in the year 993.

We tried to live as normal a life as anyone can when someone is battling cancer.

☐

About four months into his chemotherapy treatments, Jerry mentioned to his oncologist, "Dr. Blinders," that the muscles in his left leg frequently cramped and that he was having difficulty walking.

Dr. Blinders made a note in the records but said there was little he could do during the cancer treatments.

By April, seven months after being diagnosed and the full forty-six doses of chemo completed, Jerry couldn't walk half a mile without stopping to rest his feet and legs. Finally, the oncologist started to address these side effects. When he couldn't feel a pulse in Jerry's left foot or ankle, he ordered a Doppler exam.

The test result confirmed that Jerry had developed peripheral vascular disease (or PVD, also called peripheral artery disease, or PAD), which compromises circulation. Age, smoking, lack of exercise, and being overweight have a huge impact on circulation, so those factors were believed to be part of the issue. But chemotherapy is also known to impact the vascular system (veins and arteries) and was considered a likely contributor to Jerry's quickly deteriorating PVD.

Additionally, chemotherapy-induced peripheral neuropathy (CIPN) can affect walking and bring about severe pain, weakness, numbness, and tingling. CIPN is caused by certain types of chemotherapy that damage different nerves, since the chemo spreads throughout the whole body.

That made it difficult to assess whether Jerry had circulation issues, neuropathy, or both. At the very least, Jerry would require surgery to improve his circulation.

Cancer. Chemotherapy. Hospitalization. Terrible flu-like side effects. Hair loss. Painful sores in his mouth that didn't heal. Fatigue. And now subsequent issues with circulation and neuropathy that limited Jerry's ability to walk and required surgery. We continued to be positive and roll with each new development, but in the background, our altered life began to ring with echoes of *What else could go wrong?*

☐

During what we thought would be one of our last office visits to the oncologist except for yearly or biyearly checkups, Dr. Blinders mentioned that there were "a couple of small spots in Jerry's lung."

"The spots have been there since his original CT scan," he said, "but the spots are so small that I wouldn't have given them a second glance, if Jerry hadn't been diagnosed with a cancer that could metastasize to the lung."

Jerry and I exchanged a look of shock. We remembered that way back at the beginning, before we even met the oncologist, Dr. GP (general practitioner) had ordered a CT scan of Jerry's chest. Dr. Blinders had never mentioned anything about spots in Jerry's lung, at *any* point during his many months of chemo treatment.

Our oncologist didn't seem too concerned. His pen scratched a brief note in the file, then he glanced at us. "We've been keeping an eye on the spots. The good news is that they haven't grown. We can tentatively plan to biopsy them while Jerry is in the hospital having surgery to resolve his circulation issues."

Soon after that appointment, we went to meet the vascular surgeon. The vascular surgeon indicated that Jerry's circulation issues weren't critical and could wait until all his cancer issues were resolved. So, Dr. Blinders scheduled biopsies on Jerry's original abdominal mass and lung.

In the backs of our minds had been the thought, *What else could go wrong?* Now we knew. In addition to testicular cancer that had metastasized to Jerry's abdomen, it might also have metastasized to his lung.

The two of us began to feel like a pair of pinballs, bouncing from one doctor to the next, from hospital to medical office, and from test to test.

Sometimes I can't believe how naive we were, and some of the incredibly foolish mistakes that we made. This next one was a doozey.

Jerry was scheduled for the biopsy on his abdomen and lung on Wednesday, the same day that the president of the company I worked for, Dave, was flying into town for a meeting. As branch manager, I had to be there. I couldn't reschedule, and Jerry didn't feel like he could either. We were both independent, can-do people, so neither of us thought Jerry shouldn't drive himself to the hospital to have the biopsies done.

What were we thinking? Obviously, we weren't.

I attended my meeting. Dave had flown in to inform me that I was being let go. The company had merged with a company in Houston, and my duties and responsibilities would be handled out of that office.

Oddly, I'd sensed this was coming. Dave appeared baffled by my calmness and acceptance of the situation.

"It's Wednesday," I said. "Do you want me to finish out the week?"

"That would be fine," he said.

We wrapped up the details, and he left.

Just minutes after the meeting, I received a phone call from the hospital.

"Ma'am, you need to come to the hospital right away. Your husband's lung collapsed during the biopsy."

"I'll be right there." I hung up and immediately dialed Dave's mobile number.

"Dave, I can't finish out the day, and I'm not sure about finishing the week. I'm heading to the hospital. My husband just had a biopsy, and they collapsed his lung."

I quickly packed up my work things and then ran for my company van.

Later, my coworker, who had been driving Dave back to the airport when I called, asked me, "What did you say to him? I thought he was going to have a heart attack!"

Of course now, as I look back, I think it's funny, but not so much at the time.

☐

At the hospital, Jerry was in pain and having trouble breathing, two common symptoms of a collapsed lung. To make matters worse, he had to lie on a very uncomfortable ER bed in a hallway. No ER rooms were available. The hospital had wanted to admit him, but there weren't any beds available in the main part of the hospital either.

I pulled up a chair next to him in the hallway and held his hand, wanting to be able to breathe for him. Around us the place teemed with patients. The doctors and nurses gave him very little attention—and no food—for eight hours.

At that point we'd had enough. I got ahold of his doctor and emphasized that Jerry would be able to rest more comfortably at home. When his doctor made a point of disagreeing, I persisted. Finally, he relented and released him so I could take him home.

Jerry was in a lot of pain, but thankful to get out of the hospital.

Back at home, Jerry found that it hurt too much to lie down to sleep, so he slept the best he could in the recliner. Sleeping and breathing can be difficult the first few days, and the prescription for recovery is rest.

Somehow rest didn't seem likely. I'd just lost my job, and we now had a lot of adjustments to make financially. But we had never been the type of people to just sit around, so because Jerry felt up to it the next afternoon, we went to the hospital to pick up his truck.

As I said, Jerry and I were always can-do people. We got things done.

☐

Shortly after we returned from the hospital with Jerry's truck, Dr. Blinders telephoned us at home with the results of the biopsies. Jerry held the phone receiver between his ear and mine.

The good news, the doctor said, was that the biopsy on the abdominal tumor was negative. All the chemotherapy had done the job on that tumor.

The bad news was that Jerry had an active cancer in his lung.

Testicular cancer can metastasize to the lung, he said, but this wasn't metastasized testicular cancer. It was a completely different cancer.

The doctor added, "The results of the biopsy on Jerry's lung show it to be non-small cell lung cancer, more than likely from Jerry's smoking. Surgery to remove the upper lobe of his right lung will be scheduled for Monday, a few days from now."

"And there is more good news," Dr. Blinders told us, now with unmistakable excitement in his voice. "We've been watching the spots since the beginning. The good news is that they haven't grown. While the chemotherapy didn't kill the lung cancer, it contained it! I can publish that finding!"

Jerry and I looked at each other. Did Dr. Blinders seem more excited about "containing" a cancer and publishing his discovery than he was about Jerry's overall well-being?

At any rate, Jerry wouldn't need more chemotherapy, or radiation. They would cut the cancer out.

□

A second cancer. And it had been inside Jerry since this all started. We had little time to process the new development. Instead, Jerry and I started to scramble.

I'd been driving a company vehicle, but I'd been let go, so we had to buy a car before his surgery. (Isn't it always the case that when it rains it pours?) His lung collapsed on Wednesday, and we headed out to shop for a car on Friday.

Jerry was a car guy, having grown up less than half a mile from race car driver Richard Petty. No way would Jerry let me buy a car out without checking it out. To be quite honest, I wouldn't want to buy it without him, and we had to find something immediately.

Usually, when we'd go shopping for a vehicle, we'd have an idea of what we were looking for. While on our way to the first dealership, Jerry asked me, "What kind of car do you want?"

It seemed such an oddly normal conversation to be having amid the whirl of the medical chaos.

"I really don't know." I'd driven a van while the kids grew up, and I'd had a minivan for work. I hadn't paid much attention to cars in years. Besides, cars all looked pretty much the same to me. There weren't the distinctive and classic car styles we'd grown up with. "I know I don't want a van, but beyond that . . ." I shrugged.

In hindsight, we were barely functioning. The Texas day grew hot and humid, and Jerry should have been resting at home in air conditioning. I felt like a deer in the headlights, trying to figure out what kind of car I wanted to drive while also struggling to wrap my head around the lung cancer diagnosis.

Somehow we found and bought a car, a convertible—I may as well have something fun—and it rolled into our driveway that evening.

For the remainder of the weekend, besides resting, Jerry spent a lot of time sending e-mails to his employer, distributors, and customers. He excelled at anticipating problems and people's needs and wanted everything taken care of smoothly and expediently. I wrapped up all the loose ends from my job that I hadn't been able to finish while I sat with Jerry at the hospital or while we were out shopping for a car. Neither of us wanted anything hanging over our heads during the surgery and recovery.

We got everything in order before I drove Jerry to the hospital Monday morning.

Neither of us had any idea what to expect. It was a more substantial procedure than we ever anticipated. The surgery to remove the cancerous upper right lobe of Jerry's lung required a large incision. It started at the front of his rib cage, continued around his side, and went up his back to the upper inside of his shoulder blade. They had to separate his ribs to remove the lobe, and then insert two drainage tubes. His scar ran at least twenty-eight inches from end to end.

The extent of the surgery led to a very painful recovery. Jerry remained in the hospital eight days, highly sedated for four of them. When his medications were lessened, he could only talk in whispers, due to the pain.

The first words he whispered to me were, "I need a nicotine patch."

My response?

"No, you don't! The nicotine is all out of your system. If you put a patch on now, you'll reintroduce it. From now on, it's a mental battle."

That may sound like a harsh response, but it was the truth. His struggle had nothing to do with physical withdrawal from a nicotine craving but with his habits related to smoking: a cigarette after a meal, with coffee or a beer, socially, and while working on projects. Depending on the situation, he said smoking calmed him, helped him think, or just gave him something to do.

I'm happy to say Jerry smoked his last cigarette and extinguished it right before walking into the hospital the morning of his lung surgery. Thankfully, with God's help, Jerry never picked up another cigarette.

As I look back, I see that God was working in our lives even then, though we didn't fully recognize it. My ability to stay home and be there for Jerry after his surgery was an enormous blessing, because if we thought recuperating from a collapsed lung had seemed hard, it was nothing compared to having a lobe of his lung removed.

Trust me when I say "blessing" was not what I was thinking while getting laid off. I felt overwhelmed with Jerry in the hospital and with what we faced. But as I recall that time in our lives, I know God was present and watching over us. Now that knowledge helps me find peace and calm in the midst of storms.

Unfortunately, Jerry and I weren't anywhere close to the end of battling our cancer-related ordeals.

In order to ensure Jerry's future health, he needed to undergo a second surgery one month later, to remove the right testicle, the source of his first cancer. As if that weren't enough, Jerry still had the circulation issue that required surgery.

On top of all that, Jerry couldn't work like he did before cancer. And I no longer had a job.

☐

Thankfully, the delicate surgery to remove Jerry's right testicle took place on an outpatient basis. That same day, Jerry was able to come home and rest, minus one of the boys.

Again, I felt blessed to still be unemployed and at home to take care of him as he recovered.

Three and a half months following the testicular surgery—just four and a half months after having major surgery to remove a lobe of his lung—the vascular surgeon ran a tube from Jerry's femoral artery (the largest artery) in his right leg to the femoral artery in his left leg, just below the blockage. Again, Jerry had a hospital stay, this time for three days. The surgery was successful, and the circulatory fix that relieved his pain, numbness, and cramping would probably last for a good two to five years.

Finally, it seemed, after a year of cancer treatment and three major surgeries, Jerry had come through it all. Now he'd simply follow up with routine CT scans and doctor appointments to make sure the cancer didn't return.

Ever the optimists, we reiterated to our family and friends what Dr. Blinders had told us—that he'd never have given those tiny spots a second glance if Jerry hadn't had a cancer that could spread to the lungs. We had been convinced, and actually believed, the silver lining in this dark cloud was that testicular cancer had led to early detection of lung cancer—that testicular cancer had saved his life.

Jerry and I were people who generally followed the rules. We'd both been taught to respect people in positions of authority, and professionals, like doctors. Therefore, it was natural for us to unquestioningly follow doctors' orders. To be compliant. "Don't make waves." "Blessed are the peacemakers." We stayed between the lines and obediently and blindly did what the doctor said.

Yes, Jerry and I used to say that testicular cancer saved Jerry's life. But that was before the truth came to light. . . .

Chapter 3
Year 2017—The Quest for Truth:
Cancers One and Two

I've already shared with you that I initially intended this book to be simple and straightforward, but my editor challenged me to add deeper recollections, and heartfelt realism. She realized the deliberately upbeat and funny, but otherwise emotionally detached, CaringBridge blog posts covered some deep wounds.

When she asked, "Diane, what was your emotional journey?" in spring 2017, I began to realize that I had walled up nearly all my instinctive reactions. Jerry and I had determined to stay positive. The bricks of my once-solid wall began to crumble, and I became aware of the truth: I'd blocked out not only emotions, but also a lot of cancer-related memories and most of the memories that had involved intense emotional pain.

It opened me up to the most difficult, heart-wrenching two years of my life, because I had to pull those buried memories to the surface. Beyond that, to ensure accuracy of the dates and details, I had to delve into Jerry's medical records.

What I uncovered in those records left me emotionally and physically devastated.

That was the point when the neat-and-tidy story shifted, when it was hijacked, and I was sent on a tangent I'd never seen coming.

What follows is that segment of the cancer journey. The quest for truth.

□

The first time I started to look through the medical records was a Saturday night around seven.

It felt daunting to look at the five-inch stack—pages and pages of mind-numbing documents with complex medical terms. It seemed overwhelming to look at, and I expected almost nothing would come of it. Personally, I didn't think it mattered all that much to have those dates, and I didn't really want to start the process. Already I'd put it off for days. The details my editor wanted didn't seem to fit with the positive and uplifting manuscript I'd written, but if that was what she needed to help me finish . . . My attempts were half-hearted at best as I sat on the bed and started looking for the dates and information she thought she needed.

As I idly paged through the documents, I prayed that the requested details would stand out, and that I wouldn't need to go through all the papers.

All at once, ". . . marinated in chemotherapy," jumped off a page at me, followed by, "He has gained eleven pounds since I last poisoned him."

My guts twisted, and all the energy drained out of me.

After taking quite some time to gather myself together, my gaze returned to the document. I tried to wrap my head around what I was reading and who had written it. The letter was from Dr. Blinders, the oncologist, to Dr. GP, our referring physician.

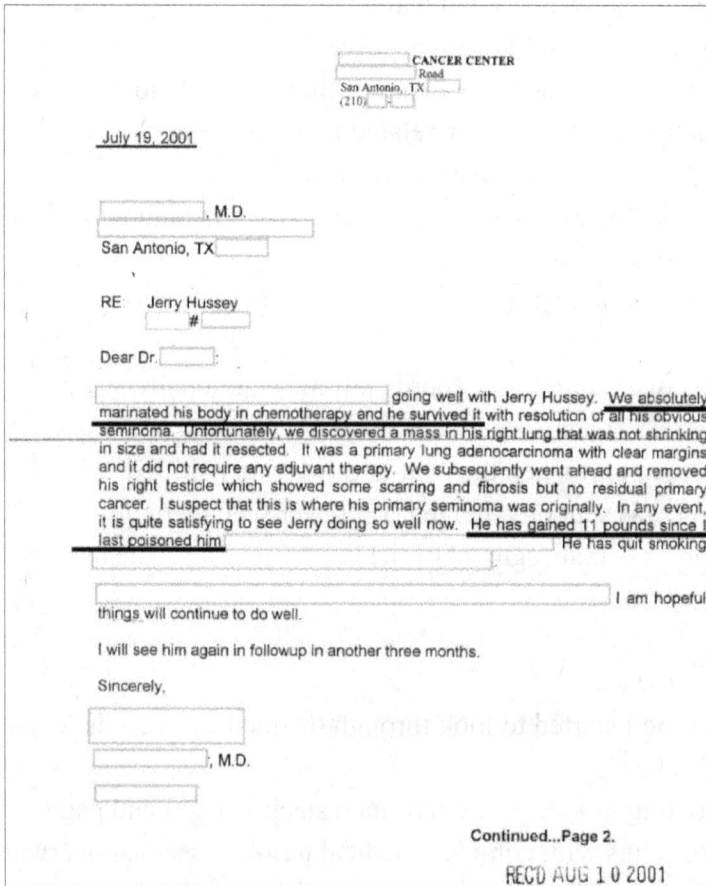

CANCER CENTER
Road
San Antonio, TX
(210)

July 19, 2001

, M.D.
San Antonio, TX

RE: Jerry Hussey
        #

Dear Dr.   :

                                                    going well with Jerry Hussey. We absolutely marinated his body in chemotherapy and he survived it with resolution of all his obvious seminoma. Unfortunately, we discovered a mass in his right lung that was not shrinking in size and had it resected. It was a primary lung adenocarcinoma with clear margins and it did not require any adjuvant therapy. We subsequently went ahead and removed his right testicle which showed some scarring and fibrosis but no residual primary cancer. I suspect that this is where his primary seminoma was originally. In any event, it is quite satisfying to see Jerry doing so well now. He has gained 11 pounds since I last poisoned him.   He has quit smoking

                                                                    I am hopeful things will continue to do well.

I will see him again in followup in another three months.

Sincerely,

                    , M.D.

Continued...Page 2.

REC'D AUG 1 0 2001

July 19, 2001, document[1]

---

[1] This and all documents, and sections of documents, included in this book are not recreations. They are photocopies of Jerry Hussey's original medical documents, with added underscores for emphasis and omissions of doctors' identifying information.

Marinated. In chemotherapy. The words pierced me and left me traumatized, weak, and sick to my stomach.

Then rage struck. I stood, started pacing, screaming, crying out in sheer agony until I found myself gasping to catch my breath.

Eventually, I made it down to the kitchen to get some comfort food and a cup of tea, to distract myself and try to calm down. Calmer but still shaken, I knew I had to go back upstairs to confront the devastating letter once again.

As I picked it up, my eyes focused on "since I last poisoned him." Yes, chemotherapy *is* poison. I understood that. But the callousness of the oncologist appalled me. I couldn't conceive of a doctor who so cavalierly talked about "poisoning" people for a living.

". . . Marinated his body in chemotherapy . . . since I last poisoned him." Those phrases swirled in my mind until they morphed to become *marinated in poison*. My stomach churned as I understood that it was an accurate description of chemotherapy.

I read the letter slowly for the first time. ". . . Marinated his body in chemotherapy *and he survived it*."

> going well with Jerry Hussey. We absolutely
> marinated his body in chemotherapy and he survived it with resolution of all his obvious

from July 19, 2001, document

What? Did the doctor *not* expect Jerry to survive all the treatment? I sat there, unable to think. Was this Dr. Blinder's attempt at humor? It disgusted and sickened me, and I was left completely shattered.

Exhausted physically, mentally, and emotionally, I needed to step away from it, needed something to distract me. No way would I be able to sleep, so I went back to the kitchen in search of something else to eat. I left the letter on the table and started cooking, hoping to settle down, but my mind continued to race. *What else might I find?!*

Oddly, the word *sifting* entered my thoughts. Along with it, I experienced a brief vision—sand and gravel being sifted through a wire mesh, the larger nuggets held by the mesh, the granules falling away below it. After a moment, the experience faded away.

It was a mystery why the word *sifting* and the vision occurred to me. However, after finding that letter from Dr. Blinders, I knew I had to get serious about going through the mound of records.

My snack consumed, I started sorting all the paperwork with determination and resolve: according to doctors and hospitals, and then chronologically. That first night I worked until 2:00 a.m., using the surface of our queen-sized bed to sort the papers.

At two o'clock, bone-weary, I knew better than to try to move anything, so I headed to the guest room to crash.

The next morning, I woke up feeling like a crazed animal. *". . . Marinated his body in chemotherapy. . . . Poisoned him."* I'd only had a few hours of sleep, but I needed to know the truth. All of it. Though it was Sunday, I didn't go to church. Instead I continued organizing and combing through the paperwork in our bedroom. Then, acknowledging that the bedroom was needed for sleeping in, I relocated the stacks to the living room couch, foyer bench, and kitchen table.

I became compulsive. I had no idea what I was looking for specifically, just that I needed to find . . . something. But what?

That same word, *sifting*, and the vision of sand and gravel being sifted, kept coming to me, like the pendulum of a grandfather clock swinging away, and then returning. Away, and back. *Sifting. Sifting.*

I sorted and read relentlessly for hours, until I couldn't work any longer. I'd worked myself into such a fog that I had no clue how much time had passed. I lay down to take a nap. When my watch went off, I couldn't understand why it was telling me to get up and exercise, to get my steps in. I thought, *That's strange. It doesn't go off this early.* But I got up, got my steps in, drank some water, and then lay back down, instantly falling back to sleep.

It happened again just before eight o'clock. My watch again reminded me it was time to get up and move. Yet outside looked like nighttime. Then I realized it was 8:00 p.m., not 8:00 a.m.—I had literally worked myself into such a state of exhaustion that I had no idea which day it was, or what time. I was literally twelve hours off.

While pondering that, I started getting the word *contrast*, paired with the words *light/dark*, *truth/lies*, and *good/evil*. They joined the refrain of *sifting* in my thoughts. Why?

I resumed reading, still unsure of what I was looking for. And then I found this—the results of the original CT scan of Jerry's chest, ordered by Dr. GP (general practitioner). It was one of the tests Jerry had completed before our first appointment with the oncologist.

```
PATIENT NAME                           ACCOUNT NO.      AGE/SEX     RADIOLOGY NUMBER
HUSSEY,JERRY                                            51/M

AT THE REQUEST OF                                       DATE OF BIRTH   DATE OF SERVICE
                      M.D.                                              09/21/2000

SAN ANTONIO, TX
```

09/21/2000: 071260 THORAX W-CON
CT EXAMINATION OF THE CHEST:

HISTORY: STOMACH MASS

FINDINGS:
Study was performed with IV contrast enhancement.

This study reveals a 3 x 2.1 cm irregular nodular density within the right apex. There is a central area of lucency within this nodule. Both lungs are otherwise clear with no additional nodules identified. No infiltrates are identified. Within the mediastinum, no mediastinal mass or adenopathy is identified.

IMPRESSION:
1.   3 CM IRREGULAR NODULAR DENSITY WITHIN THE RIGHT APEX. THIS NODULE IS INDETERMINATE AND COULD REPRESENT SCARRING, HOWEVER, CERTAINLY COULD ALSO REPRESENT TUMOR. BIOPSY SHOULD BE STRONGLY CONSIDERED.
2.   PRELIMINARY REPORT WAS CALLED TO DR.   'S OFFICE.

from September 21, 2000, document

A *3 cm mass* in Jerry's lung? *What?*

I ran to get a ruler. *How big is 3 cm?* Bigger than a quarter, I found, which is 2.5 cm. The mass was about the size of a walnut. We were told nothing about a mass!

My heart skipped a beat when I turned to this page—the radiologist's findings regarding another chest CT scan, which Dr. Blinders, the oncologist, had ordered about ten weeks into Jerry's chemo treatment.

PATIENT NAME HUSSEY, JERRY	ACCOUNT NO	AGE/SEX 51/M	RADIOLOGY NUMBER
AT THE REQUEST OF 　　　　　　 M.D. 　　　　　 DR. SAN ANTONIO, TX		DATE OF BIRTH	DATE OF SERVICE 12/04/2000

12/04/2000: 071260 THORAX W-CON
CT THORAX WITH CONTRAST:

HISTORY: SEMINOMA

COMPARISON STUDY: 9/21/00.

FINDINGS:
The spiculated right apical mass appears minimally reduced in size by several millimeters. This could be the difference in slice acquisition versus a true slight decrease in size since September.

Several very tiny 1-2 mm nodular densities in the lungs are similar to prior study and they are non-specific. No discrete pulmonary nodule in the parenchyma are identified.

No pathological mediastinal lymphadenopathy is evident.

IMPRESSION:
MINIMAL REDUCTION IN SIZE OF RIGHT APICAL SPICULATED MASS-LIKE DENSITY. THIS NOW MEASURES APPROXIMATELY 1.5 X 2 CM.

from December 4, 2000, document

Several tiny *nodular densities* in Jerry's lung? Not "spots"? I pondered. I guess spots seemed reasonable instead of Dr. Blinders speaking to us in medical jargon. But, when we first met the oncologist, he didn't even tell us about the "spots" in Jerry's lung. When he finally told us anything regarding the lung—after Jerry had completed six months of chemo—the doctor had *only* mentioned "a couple of small spots."

But there had also been a mass the size of a walnut, which the oncologist had never told us about.

This discovery felt almost surreal.

Dazed, I looked again at the original 9/21/2000, radiology report.

IMPRESSION:
1.　3 CM IRREGULAR NODULAR DENSITY WITHIN THE RIGHT APEX. THIS NODULE IS INDETERMINATE AND COULD REPRESENT SCARRING, HOWEVER, CERTAINLY COULD ALSO REPRESENT TUMOR. BIOPSY SHOULD BE STRONGLY CONSIDERED.
2.　PRELIMINARY REPORT WAS CALLED TO DR.　　　　'S OFFICE.

from September 21, 2000, document

". . . Tumor. Biopsy should be strongly considered."

The feeling of astonishment rapidly turned to anger.

Dr. Blinders had *known* Jerry likely had cancer in his lung since the very beginning, though apparently, he had assumed (wrongly) that it was metastasized testicular cancer. The only conclusion that can be drawn from this is that he blatantly lied by saying, "a couple of small spots," and by not telling us about this 3 cm tumor. *Ever.*

I stood near my office desk, ruler in hand. My mind flashed back to the oncologist's office.

I had asked him, "Since Jerry has been diagnosed with cancer, should he give up smoking cigarettes?" I'd thought, *Undoubtedly the doctor will say that he should, and Jerry will give up the two-and-a-half packs a day habit.*

The oncologist had pushed up his glasses. "No, giving it up would be too stressful."

My mind flashed back to Jerry's initial hospital stay.

During the first five days of Jerry's chemo, the kids and I had walked through the halls alongside Jerry in his hospital garb. He'd push his IV pole with its bag hanging as we headed to or from the elevator so he could go to the roof to smoke. The guys had joined their dad while Tara and I had stood at a distance since we both disliked cigarette smoke.

Setting aside the memory, I tried to process the new lung information. Was I missing something? Was I making any wrong assumptions?

Okay, I thought, *just the facts:* Dr. Blinders had known that Jerry had had an undiagnosed mass the size of a walnut in his lung for seven months before he chose to biopsy. He'd said that Jerry could continue to smoke because quitting would be too stressful, ignoring the fact that my husband had smoked two-and-a-half packs of cigarettes daily for thirty years.

Why didn't Dr. Blinders biopsy the mass to get an accurate assessment of my husband's true health condition?

The ruler trembled in my hand.

A dozen thoughts ran around in my head, but my objective reasoning joined the swarm. *Maybe Dr. Blinders had kept the truth from us so that we wouldn't experience additional worry, which might have impeded Jerry's recovery.*

Bookmarking that thought, I put the ruler down and returned to the 12/4/2000 radiologist's comparison study.

> **COMPARISON STUDY:** 9/21/00.
>
> **FINDINGS:**
> The spiculated right apical mass appears minimally reduced in size by several millimeters. This could be the difference in slice acquisition versus a true slight decrease in size since September.

from December 4, 2000, document

This chest CT scan—the one performed about ten weeks after chemotherapy began—showed that the mass, also called a nodule, was "spiculated." *And what does that mean?* I wondered.

I opened my laptop and researched the term online.

> Spiculated mass: A lump of tissue with spikes or points on the surface.[2]

Just how does that factor in? (Below, my emphases are in *italics*.)

> The radiographic edge characteristics of a pulmonary nodule *influence the probability of malignancy*. Nodule edges can be smooth, *lobulated*, irregular, and *spiculated* based on CT appearance. Typically, benign nodules have well-defined borders while malignant nodules are irregular or elongated. . . . A *spiculated* edge is an independent predictor of malignancy in a lung nodule.[3]

I rifled through records until I found the next CT scan.

PATIENT NAME HUSSEY,JERRY	ACCOUNT NO	AGE/SEX 51/M	RADIOLOGY NUMBER
AT THE REQUEST OF ___ M.D. ___ DR. SAN ANTONIO, TX		DATE OF BIRTH	DATE OF SERVICE 02/13/2001

02/13/2001: 071260 THORAX W-CON
CT OF THE CHEST:

HISTORY: TESTICULAR CANCER

FINDINGS:
Since 12/4/00, the right apical spiculated lesion now measures 2.5 x 1 cm.   Therefore, the lesion volume appears to be unchanged but it does appear to be more lobulated at this time. The remainder of the lungs are clear except for a few non-specific tiny nodules as described previously.

The mediastinum is normal.

IMPRESSION:
RIGHT APICAL SPICULATED LESION HAS A MORE LOBULATED APPEARANCE AT THIS TIME, EVEN THOUGH THIS MAY BE DUE TO TECHNIQUE SUCH AS SLICE SELECTION. FOLLOW-UP CT IS RECOMMENDED, OR ALTERNATIVELY A PET SCAN MAY BE OBTAINED.

from February 13, 2001, document

---

[2] https://www.cancer.gov/publications/dictionaries/cancer-terms?cdrid=44505
[3] http://www.clevelandclinicmeded.com/medicalpubs/diseasemanagement/hematology-oncology/pulmonary-nodules/

Lobulated. More lobes had formed on the lung mass in the two months since the previous CT scan. And lobulated meant *likelihood of cancer.*

I again felt sickened to think that for seven months the oncologist had ignored the recommendation to biopsy and ignored the subsequent CT scans that indicated Jerry had a sizable cancerous mass in his lung.

Along with testicular cancer, Jerry had also had a second form of the disease—lung cancer.

It seemed clear the oncologist had been laying odds that the testicular cancer had metastasized to the lung, so he didn't follow up on the recommendation to biopsy to find out whether he was actually dealing with one form of cancer or two (thus cementing my name for him, Dr. Blinders).

Remember how I said that we'd told our family and friends we'd felt the silver lining in the dark cloud was that testicular cancer had saved Jerry's life, due to the lung cancer being discovered at a relatively early stage? In truth it had been discovered seven months before we were told anything about it. In addition, the lung cancer had existed to a degree that we had never known, until I learned about it in the medical records seventeen years later.

And Dr. Blinders had left the lung cancer to remain, and Jerry had been left to smoke.

Standing in our living room, recalling the day we had received Dr. Blinders' phone call telling us about the second cancer, it was all I could do not to fling the documents across the room.

If that wasn't bad enough, I was stopped cold with recalling the excitement in Dr. Blinders' voice when he'd said, "While the chemotherapy didn't kill the lung cancer, it contained it! I can publish that finding." In essence he had patted himself on the back for preventing growth of the lung cancer temporarily. He had considered his actions a job well done. Jerry and I both had been left with the distinct impression that Dr. Blinders had seemed more excited about "containing" a cancer and publishing his findings than he had been about Jerry's overall well-being.

Now I had a good idea why: The oncologist had been excited about "containing" the lung cancer because he'd had a heart-clenching "oh-crap" moment when he discovered that the lung held a second cancer, lung cancer, and not a metastasis of testicular cancer as he'd thought. The upper right lobe of Jerry's lung had been removed just five days after he'd ordered the biopsy.

Enraged that he had withheld critical information from us from the beginning—information that would likely have caused Dr. Blinders to reevaluate how to treat the two different cancers had we all known about it—

and that he'd made an assumption about the type of cancer in Jerry's lung—a wrong assumption—I vacillated from anger and rage to crumbling and crying.

Finally, I felt empty. But it wasn't my nature to remain that way for long. What would that accomplish? A resolve to find the truth took root far within. I knew I had to become a detective and sift through all the unknowns. I needed answers.

☐

Returning to the documents, I dug in again. Was there anything else we hadn't known at the time?

> IMPRESSION:
> RIGHT APICAL SPICULATED LESION HAS A MORE LOBULATED APPEARANCE AT THIS TIME, EVEN THOUGH THIS MAY BE DUE TO TECHNIQUE SUCH AS SLICE SELECTION. FOLLOW-UP CT IS RECOMMENDED, OR ALTERNATIVELY A PET SCAN MAY BE OBTAINED.

from February 13, 2001, document

Oh, wow. The 2/13/2001 radiologist's results, from five months into Jerry's first chemotherapy, had included the recommendation that the oncologist confirm with a follow-up CT, or perform a PET (positron emission tomography) scan.

A PET scan, I now know, will detect cancer wherever it shows up in the body.[4] (Below, my clarifications are in parentheses.)

> During a PET scan, the patient is first injected with a glucose (sugar) solution that contains a very small amount of radioactive material. The substance is absorbed by the particular organs or tissues being examined. The patient rests on a table and slides into a large tunnel-shaped scanner. The PET scanner is then able to "see" damaged or cancerous cells where the glucose is being taken up (cancer cells often use more glucose than normal cells) and the rate at which the tumor is using the glucose (which can help determine the tumor grade). . . .
>
> A PET scan can be used to detect cancerous tissues and cells in the body that may not always be found through computed tomography (CT) or magnetic resonance imaging (MRI).[5]

---

[4] Note that PET scans do not detect every form of cancer.

> PET scans can reveal the presence and stage of a cancer,
> show whether and where it has spread, and help doctors decide
> on treatment. A PET scan can give an idea of how well
> chemotherapy is working, and it can detect a recurring tumor
> sooner than other techniques.[6]

PET scans have been used routinely since the 1990s, so there wasn't any logical reason that the oncologist hadn't ordered the PET scan. With Jerry's two-and-a-half packs a day cigarette habit over thirty years, wouldn't you think Dr. Blinders would have seen the need to find out whether the mass and nodules were a result of metastatic testicular cancer OR actually lung cancer as a result of decades of smoking?

I sifted through the stack of paperwork again, and again. Each time, I started down a new trail and had to look up all the medical jargon to understand the terminology. I not only wanted to understand it for myself, but if I found anything to share, it needed to be understandable. Even as I researched each detail to the nth degree, I still knew I was missing something.

Eventually, months later, I found it.

Hypercalcemia shows up in Jerry's initial paperwork from Dr. Blinders for cancer one, but it actually became the last piece of the puzzle in the many months of researching all of his cancers. I'd looked up every other medical term, I believe, and now felt prompted to look up this word. Once I'd researched hypercalcemia, and then calmed down, I knew I'd found the final piece.

The word appeared in a September 27, 2000, letter. It was the first letter from the oncologist, Dr. Blinders, to Dr. GP, as Jerry's cancer treatment began.

---

[5] https://www.cancercenter.com/treatments/pet-scan/
[6] https://www.medicalnewstoday.com/articles/154877.php

CANCER CENTER
Rd.
San Antonio, TX
(210) -

September 27, 2000

, M.D.
Dr. #
San Antonio, TX

RE: Jerry Hussey

Dear Dr.   :

Thank you very much for letting me become involved in the care of Jerry Hussey. The final pathology revealed seminoma. He may have a primary in the right testicle. On the other hand, his massive retroperitoneal involvement has not allowed me the luxury of definitively diagnosing his right testicle abnormality. We have admitted him to the _____ Hospital where we have initiated treatment with a combination of carboplatin and VP-16. He also had hypercalcemia and was given pamidronate and IV fluids with normal saline and furosemide for this problem. Hopefully he will have a good outcome from this therapy.

I very much appreciate the opportunity of participating in his care.

Sincerely,

, M.D.

RECD OCT 0 9 2000

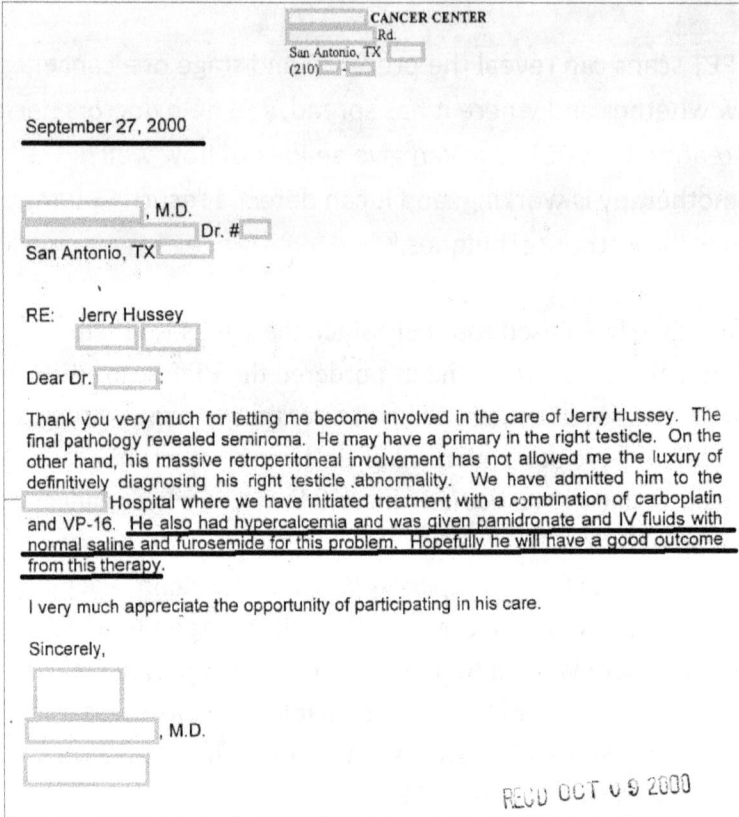

September 27, 2000, document

And what is hypercalcemia?

> An increased level of calcium in the bloodstream is most often a complication of cancer and is referred to as hypercalcemia of malignancy. In its severe form, hypercalcemia may be a life-threatening emergency.[7]

Life-threatening emergency? My heart started to race. I read further, needing to know and understand now what we hadn't been told then. (My emphases are in *italics*.)

---

[7] https://www.mayoclinic.org/diseases-conditions/hypercalcemia/symptoms-causes/syc-20355523

Hypercalcemia is caused by . . .

- **Cancer.** *Lung* cancer and breast cancer, as well as some cancers of the blood, can increase your risk of hypercalcemia.[8]

Hypercalcemia of malignancy occurs in approximately 10 percent of patients with advanced cancers. The occurrence of hypercalcemia may rise as high as 40 percent in some types of cancer, including breast, *lung*, and multiple myeloma. . . .

This disorder can be severe and difficult to manage. . . .

In a person with cancer, a high blood calcium level is considered a medical emergency and treatment should be started immediately.[9]

Up to 20 percent of individuals with cancer will develop hypercalcemia at some point in their disease.[10]

If hypercalcemia is seen in the presence of cancer, the average 30-day survival rate is about 50 percent.[11]

What?! I was stunned and reread the line: "If hypercalcemia is seen in the presence of cancer, the average 30-day survival rate is about 50 percent." And we were never told? We were *never told*! Those are not good odds. Dr. Blinders had quoted the success rate with testicular cancer as 95 percent, and we had been content with those odds. But he'd never disclosed Jerry's hypercalcemia or his 50/50 chances.

Now, honestly, based on that information, it should have been imperative that the doctor share the seriousness of the situation. Instead of spending the weekend getting caught up on details for our employers, perhaps Jerry and I should have been making sure his will and his other legal affairs were in order.

Astounded, I reread and pondered the rest of the information and implications of the articles. I also found this. (My clarification is in parentheses and emphasis is in *italics*.)

---

[8] https://www.mayoclinic.org/diseases-conditions/hypercalcemia/symptoms-causes/syc-20355523

[9] http://news.cancerconnect.com/types-of-cancer/bone-cancer/hypercalcemia/

[10] https://answers.webmd.com/answers/1178124/what-are-the-causes-of-hypercalcemia

[11] https://www.medicinenet.com/hypercalcemia/article.htm

Seminomas (testicular cancer) have been *rarely* associated
with malignant hypercalcemia.[12]

So, hypercalcemia can result from *lung* cancer, but *rarely* from testicular cancer. That should have been a big, red flag for the oncologist from the get-go.

Hypercalcemia had been one of Jerry's high-priority issues that had put him in the hospital for his first round of chemo. We really hadn't understood at the time why Jerry needed to be hospitalized, because most people have chemo as outpatients. But hypercalcemia is considered a medical emergency in someone with cancer. Yet we hadn't asked questions. Our response had been Pavlovian. We had just gone along with what the doctor had said.

Had Dr. Blinders kept the truth from us so that we wouldn't experience additional worry?

To answer that for myself, I listed the information Dr. Blinders had kept from us and include it here to document our objectivity.

- On 9/21/2000 the chest CT scan ordered by Dr. GP (general practitioner) revealed a 3 cm mass in Jerry's lung. In his report, the CT scan radiologist noted, "tumor. Biopsy should be strongly considered." The CT scan radiologist had been so alert to the implications that he had chosen to call the doctor's office to verbally convey the preliminary report.
- On 12/4/2000 the chest CT scan radiologist, in his report, noted to Dr. Blinders that the lung mass was "spiculated." My research revealed, "A spiculated edge is an independent predictor of malignancy in a lung nodule."
- On 2/13/2001 the chest CT scan radiologist, in his report, noted to Dr. Blinders, "Right apical spiculated lesion has a *more lobulated* appearance." My research revealed that lobulated meant likelihood of cancer. The CT scan radiologist, in his report, noted to Dr. Blinders, "Follow-up CT is recommended, or alternatively a PET scan may be obtained."
- Going back to 9/27/2000, Dr. Blinders, in his own letter to Dr. GP, noted, "He also had hypercalcemia." My research revealed, "*Lung* cancer and breast cancer, as well as some cancers of the blood, can

---

[12] https://www.ncbi.nlm.nih.gov/pmc/articles/PMC3991903/

increase your risk of hypercalcemia." Lung cancer is specified in relation to hypercalcemia, whereas a testicular-cancer relation is rare.

Dr. Blinders had:

- ignored the radiologist's 9/21/2000 recommendation to biopsy the lung nodule.
- ignored the radiologist's 2/13/2001 recommendation to obtain a follow-up CT or PET scan of the lung nodule.
- ignored the science behind his own diagnosis of hypercalcemia, that it occurs most notably in patients with lung cancer as opposed to testicular cancer.
- biopsied the lung seven months after the initial 9/21/2000 radiologist's recommendation to biopsy.
- discovered via biopsy that the walnut-sized lung nodule was a second form of cancer.
- had the cancerous upper right lobe of Jerry's lung surgically removed just five days after the biopsy revealed the second form of cancer, pretty fast action for a cancer that the doctor had repeatedly ignored.

Additional observations of Dr. Blinders.

→ He never told us about the hypercalcemia.
→ He never told us about the sizable cancerous mass/tumor in Jerry's lung.
→ He'd said, "The spots have been there since his original CT scan, but the spots are so small that I wouldn't have given them a second glance, if Jerry hadn't been diagnosed with a cancer that could metastasize to the lung." So he'd believed that the cancer in the lung had been metastasized testicular cancer.
→ Jerry and I both had been left with the distinct impression Dr. Blinders had seemed more excited about "containing" a cancer than he was about Jerry's overall well-being. It had sounded strongly like relief.
→ All available indicators point to the conclusion that Dr. Blinders had wrongly lain odds that the cancer in the lung was metastasized testicular cancer that would be largely eliminated by the chemotherapy, when in fact it had been a second, concurrent, cancer. This was information that likely would have led the doctor to take different action, including encouraging Jerry to quit smoking. As for Jerry and me, we would have

compliantly gone with whatever treatment we were told. The onus was on the doctor to act based on the information he had received from all the test results that he'd received, as well as Jerry's health history, which included his smoking habit.

With these factors objectively considered, Dr. Blinders' actions indicated negligence beyond keeping a patient and their family from worry by means of adjusting the truth. He'd made mistakes and covered them up. He had blatantly withheld potentially life-and-death medical information about hypercalcemia and what was ultimately proven to be lung cancer.

In hindsight, I wish we'd pursued the world of alternative cancer therapies early on, but honestly, I don't know what options may have been available at that time. We certainly weren't aware of any alternatives to conventional treatment.

□

I had to take a break for days to clear my head and circle back around to process all the information one more time.

To recap, Dr. Blinder's course of treatment had been chemotherapy for the first cancer, followed by surgery to remove a lobe of Jerry's right lung for the second cancer, and then removal of the right testicle (the first cancer).

I wanted to give grace to Dr. Blinders for his errors, yet my thoughts were churning in two directions. *What if we give the doctor the benefit of the doubt, and consider that he'd made a mistake? We are all human, and we all make mistakes.*

But this is more than a mistake. With all the test results and documentation, it's apparent that there was an attempt to cover up, and evidence that my husband's health was not Dr. Blinder's first and foremost concern.

I believe Dr. Blinders' communication to us, both his lack of disclosure and his understating the facts, had been unconscionable. At the very beginning we should have been told the truth—yes, in a way that wouldn't incite panic—and the lung biopsy and PET scan should have been performed.

I have no tolerance for lies, which makes this all the more painful to me. We bought into the lie—that Dr. Blinders wouldn't have given the spots a second glance if it hadn't been for the fact that Jerry had a cancer that could metastasize to his lung. We became a party to the lie, telling everyone that the silver lining in the dark cloud was that testicular cancer had saved Jerry's life.

Now I had learned the truth.

Thankfully we have the copies of Jerry's medical records so that we don't have to subjectively look at the nightmare of the journey through my recollections. We can objectively look at the hell of cancer as documented by doctors and test results. My conclusion: This is an indictment of an oncologist who failed us. And, I'm sorry to say, he would not be the only one.

Chapter 4
Cancer Three

San Antonio, Texas
January 2002

Jerry's two cancers and medical odyssey had taken up a year of our lives. The surgery to resolve his circulation issue had been completed in September 2001. He'd slowly been able to resume visiting his customers and traveling to see his distributors. Our lives were finally becoming normal again.

From the time Jerry's lung cancer was diagnosed, actually from the day they collapsed his lung and I lost my job, I was unemployed. One positive that resulted, in addition to being there for Jerry as he went through his surgeries and medical issues, was that I'd been receiving unemployment. While that didn't come close to my salary, at least we had something coming in.

Between being with Jerry during his surgeries and caring for him as he recovered, I dutifully looked for a job. However, the job market at the time wasn't very good in San Antonio, and I wasn't able to find work.

In January 2002, my unemployment was running out. I needed to find *something*. You know how desperate people do desperate things? I responded to an ad—to sell cars. (You've got to love the humor here, since I'd had no clue what kind of car I'd wanted eight months prior!) The deal was that I would receive one week of training at a cost of $549. If I was still employed at the end of ninety days, I would receive my money back. If not, I'd lose it all.

Now, how many people go out and "buy" a job? Although the idea sounded a little crazy, the bills were piling up, and the job market remained abysmal.

And, as the dealership explained, anyone who learned how to sell cars would always be able to find a job. They'd found that the turnover rate decreased, and their salespeople were far more committed, when they first invested in themselves financially via the training program.

Three of the ten in our class were women. At the time, the company didn't have any women salespeople. The salesmen already working for the dealership had a bet: Who would be the first one to quit? Nearly all of them picked me, and so the payoff would come with who was closest to the date I would throw in the towel.

Little did they realize how tenacious (and cheap) I could be. I was not about to quit on myself or our money. Actually, the first one to quit had convinced management that he was a sales star and didn't need to take the class. Nobody picked him to quit first, but it seemed the dealership was right—there was no commitment, and he was the first one to leave.

I never achieved the rank of top salesperson but could always be found in the top half. Unlike most of the salespeople at that dealership, I always treated customers how I liked to be treated, or how I hoped a car salesperson would take care of my parents or my kids. Car salespeople had a terrible reputation (often deservedly so), and they would gloat as they bragged about "knocking their heads off," meaning they'd scored a huge commission. My goal was to treat people truthfully and fairly. For me, it was a real learning experience from all sides—management, the sales team, and customers.

☐

In August 2002, Jerry lost his job. It had been almost a year since Jerry had undergone his final medical procedure to improve his circulation, and nearly two years since he had been diagnosed with his first cancer. We both believed he was let go because of the cancer diagnosis, and that his employers had waited what they thought was a "respectable amount" of time before firing him.

It made no sense whatsoever. It wasn't that he couldn't do his job. While going through cancer treatment, Jerry remained more than 10 percent over goal, in spite of his limited ability to travel and make sales calls in person. He supported his customers and distributors through e-mails and phone calls, and kept his employer apprised of everything.

Furthermore, Jerry always had a strong work ethic and was a loyal employee. His customers and distributors respected and liked Jerry, and his sales numbers showed it.

We could only surmise that the company had determined that because he'd had cancer, Jerry had become an uncertain element, one that might possibly develop cancer again. A liability, and they weren't about to take a chance. (Jerry remained friends with several people in the company, as well as his distributors, and he smiled as he heard that his replacements always fell far short and never lasted long.)

It wasn't fair, so Jerry went to an attorney. But his employer was in a right-to-work state and firing him was legal. Jerry had been highly sought after in his field, often contacted by recruiters. But his industry was tight-knit and well-connected. Doors that had previously been open for him were now closed, simply because of the cancer diagnosis. Jerry couldn't find a job in Texas, or anywhere else in that industry. I include this only to say that people who have or had cancer face huge challenges in more areas than just health.

Jerry had had a long and successful work history but now encountered the same difficulties I'd had in trying to find a job. Week after week he looked locally. We really wanted to stay in San Antonio.

Personally, I thought he would do well selling cars. I mean, if I could do it . . . He was an excellent salesman and knew a lot about cars. He could talk up one side and down the other about cars from the '50s, '60s, and '70s but, like me, thought most of the current cars looked similar and were boring.

He enjoyed industrial sales and had no desire to deal with the general public, and he'd probably heard far too many complaints about car sales from me.

Rather than stew in frustration, Jerry and I asked each other, "Well then, what *can* we do?" As we brainstormed possibilities, we talked about moving back to Chicago. My parents were in their seventies, and it made sense to be near them. Jerry started exploring Illinois-based industrial sales jobs outside the field that he'd worked in for nearly thirty years. Fortunately he found a company that recognized his abilities, with a huge territory that included the midwestern states, from Texas to Illinois and beyond. It was a good fit. Jerry could go to Illinois, work the territory while looking for a new home, and we could move our household when the time was right.

In the interim, we started preparing our home for sale. We rid the house of clutter and did everything our realtor recommended.

On a Thursday, we listed our house in San Antonio. On Friday, our daughter, Tara, graduated from Air Force basic training, and we spent the weekend enjoying her company, knowing that we wouldn't be seeing her all that often anymore. The following Monday, Tara left for training in northern Texas, and Jerry left for a sales trip in Illinois. On Tuesday, we had three offers for the house, and got our full asking price.

☐

At my job, the dealership environment had deteriorated rapidly after about a year. One of my female classmates quit and filed a sexual harassment complaint with human resources, and HR called me in to describe the work environment and what I had perceived and experienced.

Someone obviously leaked my being questioned by HR to the sales manager, "Bob," or his dad, who was the vice president. Bob believed himself untouchable in his position. I was called into Bob's office, a glass cubicle in the corner of the showroom, where he berated me for what I had told the HR manager. I stood there receiving his insults. I didn't get upset or emotional, which made Bob all the angrier.

Finally, nearly shouting, he exclaimed, "I'd rather go down for hitting a woman on the showroom floor than for an allegation of sexual harassment."

Needless to say, many people witnessed the incident, and Bob was relieved of his position. It really didn't matter to me. I was putting in my resignation because Jerry and I would be moving back to Illinois.

No, I wasn't the first, second, or even third to quit the car business. For fifteen months I'd sold cars in the Texas heat (and mild winters) before moving on. And I was the last of the three women standing.

While it wasn't my favorite job, it had paid the bills and helped us catch up on some expenses. The experience was valuable, and soon the trainer would be proven correct: Once you learn how to sell cars, you'll always be able to get a job.

☐

Jerry arrived in northeastern Illinois and immediately went from house hunting to house buying. We'd made a list of all we wanted in a home, and he found something close and put in an offer. The owners were said to be absolutely firm on their price, but, of course, we offered less.

Most people couldn't believe that I was fine with Jerry buying the house alone, and that I didn't see the house until the day before closing at the walkthrough. We'd been married more than thirty years, and I trusted Jerry's judgment. But even more than that, I believed I'd heard God give me a price. That was what we offered, and it was accepted. I felt at peace the whole time, knowing God was in control.

☐

Northeastern Illinois
Summer 2003

As soon as we settled in our new Illinois home, Jerry went to visit his new oncologist (whom I will call "Dr. Lance" for reasons that will be revealed). Jerry had all of Dr. Blinder's records from San Antonio transferred. We liked Dr. Lance well enough—while all was well.

I started working part-time as a caregiver. I really enjoyed helping people while I tried to figure out what I wanted to do. I didn't want to go into accounting, even though I had my degree, and just didn't want to get into a large corporate environment. I was fifty years old and hadn't figured out what to be when I grew up.

Life was good. Jerry had started doing woodworking in San Antonio, and he expanded his woodworking shop in his new garage. One of the requirements for our home had been an attached garage for me and a detached garage for Jerry's shop. We didn't get all the things we'd hoped for in a home, but we did get the garages.

We had a great time building his woodshop. We planned it out, insulated it, put in a dust-collection system, built workbenches, and installed a heater. He could work comfortably year-round, even with below-zero Midwestern winters.

Jerry enjoyed making custom furniture for our home—bedroom and living room, plus bookshelves, coat racks, various gifts, and most especially decorative boxes with hinged lids to hold mementos. He never made two pieces alike and wouldn't use screws or nails except for the hinges. He was truly a craftsman and an artist. Occasionally he sold some pieces, but more often than not, he gave them away to friends or others who enjoyed this creative part of him.

About a year after we settled into our home, the company that had brought us to Chicago was sold and reorganized, and Jerry was let go. Though he'd already become the top regional manager, it didn't matter because he'd been with the company for the shortest time.

I needed to find a full-time job with benefits, so I went back to selling cars. Again, the salesmen bet that I wouldn't make it more than a few weeks, but as before I not only outlasted their expectations, I finished each month in the top half with units sold.

Jerry had trouble finding a job, which puzzled us. Finally, we had to admit that he had turned fifty-five, and age discrimination is real. Since he hated being unemployed and stagnant, he was open to any type of job. So, after thirty-plus years in sales, he obtained his CDL license and got a job driving a truck locally.

My flannel-loving Jerry was now a truckdriver.

It wasn't such a stretch of the imagination. Jerry loved to drive, and I don't believe he ever became involved in an accident as an adult. At his high school, seniors had been recruited to drive the school buses. It was hard for me to believe, since Jerry had been 5' 3" when he'd graduated from high school, and many of the kids on his bus had been taller than him. Today, it's difficult to conceive that a school district would entrust the school buses and lives of the children to high school seniors. But it's a testimony to the character of Jerry and his friends, as well as to an era where young adults were trusted with significant responsibility.

As I mentioned previously, Jerry grew up a half mile (as the crow flies) from NASCAR Hall of Famer Richard Petty. Petty is known as "The King" and is the most decorated driver in the history of NASCAR with a career record 200 wins.

Of course, Jerry and his friends had driven under the influence of young Richard, and Jerry often talked about his own driving escapades. Because he'd looked like he was about twelve years old when he'd gotten his license, he'd been stopped more than 130 times for driving underage, but he'd been legal and had never gotten a ticket.

Jerry told me he could turn his mom's 1954 VW Beetle 180 degrees in the road and drive in the opposite direction without stopping—by downshifting, turning the wheel, and pulling up the emergency brake.

When I first met Jerry, and for the first few years of our marriage, I swear I put dents in his passenger floorboard trying to help him stop the car. He drove with purpose from the time he took off until he came to a screeching halt.

Now he was driving a truck.

☐

January 2005

Nearly two years went by uneventfully. Then Jerry caught a cold, in January 2005. In addition to the regular cold symptoms, he was bothered by a noticeable and annoying stiffness that developed in his neck. Six weeks later, he still had the stiffness plus some swelling, low on the right side of his neck. We didn't want to overreact to every illness, but six weeks seemed a bit long, so he went to our family doctor, "Dr. GP 2." Based on Jerry's cancer history, the doctor recommended that he make an appointment with his oncologist.

In March Jerry went to see his oncologist, Dr. Lance. Ever the optimists, we didn't think there was anything to be overly concerned about, and Jerry worked the oncologist appointment into his schedule. Neither of us thought I needed to go to what we believed would be a routine appointment.

Dr. Lance probed the swelling in his neck and ordered numerous tests, including a CT scan. It confirmed that Jerry had a mass in the lower right region of his neck, so the doctor ordered a PET scan.

A PET scan shows whether cancer is present, and wherever it appears in the body. To reiterate, in layman's terms, a PET scan (positron emission tomography) detects the presence and severity of an active cancer. How does it do that? Before the scan, the patient receives an intravenous injection of radioactive glucose (sugar). Cancer cells *love* sugar and go into a feeding frenzy. The PET scan basically lights up to show the location, tumor size, and it differentiates cancer from benign growths.

The day after the PET scan, Dr. Lance telephoned Jerry with the results. It confirmed that the mass seen in the CT scan was, in fact, cancerous.

That night, our discussion grew somber as Jerry told me the results. We couldn't believe he had another cancer. Though we struggled to comprehend the new development, we were good for each other and good together. We knew what to say, and what not to say. We didn't have to fill the silence, but eventually one of us would find something encouraging to say. And of course, there is nothing like being held and comforted by the love of your life.

We always hear early detection is the key, so being the eternal optimists, we felt it good news that the cancer was limited to one lymph node in the neck. The bad news, in our opinion, was that it had entered the lymph system. We chose to focus on the positive. Jerry had already beaten it twice, and he'd beat it again.

Dr. Lance ordered a biopsy to determine the type of cancer and course of treatment.

The biopsy went uneventfully, and a few days later we headed to the oncologist's office for the results. I rarely went to Jerry's appointments. He always worked them into his schedule, and the doctor's office sat more than an hour's drive away. However, since we'd be discovering which kind of cancer was in Jerry's lymph node and the proposed treatment, we both agreed I needed to be there.

Jerry and I arrived and took seats in the lobby. There we watched a large aquarium of fish that reminded us of Chemo, the reddish-purple betta fish that our daughter, Tara, had bought for Jerry during his first cancer treatment. Today the fish weren't as soothing.

When called, we went to the exam room where a nurse took Jerry's vital signs. She recorded the information and left.

Dr. Lance strolled in and shut the door. "We've been unable to determine which type of cancer this is. One report indicates it's a recurrence of your testicular cancer, while another suggests lung cancer."

I'm sure he rambled on a bit as to why there was a discrepancy, but my mind wandered. I couldn't fathom why the biopsy didn't provide a clear-cut answer. I shook off the confusion to focus on the doctor's words.

". . . So, you have three options. One, we can treat it as lung cancer. Two, we can treat it as testicular cancer, through me. Or three, we can treat it as testicular cancer through Lance Armstrong's doctors." Dr. Lance nodded with enthusiasm at the third option, as if encouraging us toward that choice.

We knew that Lance Armstrong, the world-famous racing cyclist, had been diagnosed with testicular cancer in 1996. It had been considered potentially fatal since it had metastasized (spread). An inspiration to all cancer patients and survivors, Lance remained held in very high regard as he battled back from his cancer to win the Tour de France seven times from 1998 to 2005. (Since then, Lance Armstrong has fallen from grace and been stripped of his titles and achievements due to doping, but back in 2005 he gave us, and many others, hope.)

So, as Jerry learned of his third cancer, Lance Armstrong and his team of doctors remained highly respected. But we felt confused. Why was Jerry's oncologist talking to us about Lance and his doctors when he, himself, couldn't even say what kind of cancer Jerry had? It just didn't make sense.

Jerry and I exchanged looks, but we didn't need to in order to know each other's reaction: *This guy is the oncologist, and **he** is asking **us** to **guess** which kind of cancer it is . . . and how it should be treated?! We are supposed to guess? He's the doctor. He should be giving us the recommendation!*

I forced my whirling thoughts to slow down. It seemed the oncologist wanted to treat this as testicular cancer, even though he said the tests were inconclusive. My confusion returned. *Why hadn't the biopsy revealed the kind of cancer? That's what biopsies are for!*

As the discussion continued, the doctor seemed increasingly eager to refer us to the doctors that Lance Armstrong had gone to. (Thus, the name Dr. Lance.)

My thoughts took off again. He was an oncologist! Why couldn't he figure out what kind of cancer Jerry had? And why was he suggesting *we* pick a treatment, even though none of us knew what type of cancer? The whole situation seemed crazy. I was now deeply skeptical of this doctor's ability to treat my Jerry.

Jerry leaned his elbows on his knees and looked over at the Lance fan in the lab coat. "You're the doctor, and you want *us* to *guess*?"

Crickets.

In the brief silence, my mind shifted to the cancer-recurrence scenario. Why had the cancer reappeared?

As I focused and prayed to God for understanding, I had a vision of a beautiful green lawn, totally free of dandelions. Then suddenly, out of nowhere, up springs a dandelion. How did it get there? Well, it started as a seed that sprouted when the conditions were right.

Next, I envisioned a yard with dandelions popping up by the dozens, until thousands of them carpeted the yard. Then I envisioned them being sprayed with weed killer and withering and dying.

Although a lawn may be dandelion-free for a time, invariably they come back.

I said to the oncologist, "I'm trying to create a scenario to understand why Jerry's cancer has returned. Of course, I'm generalizing, comparing dandelions to cancer. So, tell me if this is a good analogy."

I reiterated the vision of the lawn covered with dandelions. I described spraying weed killer on the lawn, and that the dandelions then shrivel and die. "So, the chemo—which is poison, like the weed killer—kills the active cancer (the weeds) but does nothing to the potential cancer cells (the seeds). Then, when the conditions are right, the seeds germinate and grow. You might not notice the weeds until they start blooming again. It may take a while, even years before the cancer reappears, but when it does, it shows up like the bright yellow dandelions on a PET scan."

The doctor said, "That's a great analogy! Yes!"

"So, chemo only kills active cancer, but does nothing to prevent future recurrence."

"That's right," he agreed. "Excellent way to put it."

It was helpful to see that in my mind and understand that basic principle. But then why had I been the one to think of it? Judging by Jerry's expression, he and I both felt that the doctor should have been able to give us a better understanding about cancer and why it recurs, instead of saying nothing about it at all.

The oncologist's three options for treatment hung almost tangibly in the middle of the room.

Jerry said, "We'll need some time to think about those three choices. We're not equipped to make that decision now." His voice was polite, but flat.

Jerry and I left the office without taking a second look at the fish tank. We both agreed that we needed to get a second opinion. The two of us had a lot to talk about on our drive home, and we decided that we could not—and would not—entrust Jerry's life or health to Dr. Lance.

Within a few days we'd located a new oncologist and made an appointment.

I continued to think about the dandelion scenario. If poison (chemo) couldn't kill the seeds that grew the weeds (cancer), why weren't oncologists trying to prevent the seeds from germinating and growing?

Did they even know how to prevent cancer?

If they didn't, then was it possible that somebody else knew?

Chapter 5
Second Opinion

Bad news travels fast, especially when you find out that you have cancer and need an oncologist. There is no shortage of family and good friends who know someone who has been down that road.

Jerry's friend's mother had been treated for cancer. He remembered that his friend "Joe" had been very involved and supportive of his mother's treatment, often taking her to her doctor appointments and chemo infusions. Jerry gave him a call to find out how his mother was doing, and what he thought of the oncologist.

Joe's mother had overcome her cancer, and Joe couldn't have been more pleased. He highly recommended his mother's oncologist, who was well respected, supposedly among the top ten oncologists in the Chicagoland area.

Jerry and I headed to the first appointment with this referred oncologist, "Dr. PM," as I would soon think of him. During this appointment, we would basically interview each other—did he want Jerry as a patient, and did Jerry/we want him as Jerry's doctor?

The doctor had us brought into his eclectically decorated office. It was packed with books and Chinese artifacts, plus a large geode and a picture of his family. He seemed to be a collector of things that were given to him, perhaps by his children.

He had a calming yet highly professional demeanor, which was 180 degrees opposite of his office space. He knew we had come for a second opinion, so he asked Jerry what was going on.

Jerry outlined his cancer history—testicular and lung cancers—the types of chemotherapies received, and surgeries.

Then Jerry recounted our appointment with Dr. Lance, including the results of the CT and PET scans and biopsy. It was almost comical as Jerry discussed the inconclusive test results, and the odd way Dr. Lance had presented the three treatment options.

Dr. PM patiently listened, furrowing his brow at the treatment options. Then he told us how he would proceed if we chose to work with him, in a way that inspired our confidence. Dr. PM stated that he belonged to a group of thirteen colleagues who routinely met to review difficult and puzzling cases. He would review Jerry's records, bring them to the group, and afterward meet with us to discuss the treatment plan.

Dr. PM's professionalism and demeanor was a far cry from what we had just experienced with Dr. Lance, and we felt certain that Dr. PM was a good choice.

Dr. PM asked us to get copies of Jerry's medical records from Dr. Lance's office and bring them to him as soon as possible so that he could review them and take them to his colleagues. Once he'd had the chance to review them, he said, then he'd know how best to treat Jerry's lymph node cancer.

☐

As we left Dr. PM's office, Jerry called Dr. Lance's office to request copies of his medical records. Surprisingly, Dr. Lance and his staff took great offense that we would seek another opinion. All of Jerry's records from San Antonio had been forwarded to them, and when Jerry requested the records, he was told that the records were their property, and we couldn't have them.

Jerry had the phone on speaker, and I could hear the discussion back and forth. Unbelievably, Dr. Lance's staff sounded almost combative. Finally, Jerry threatened to have an attorney get involved. He *needed* copies of his medical records for treatment. His health and life were at stake. What good were Jerry's records to the former oncologist since he wouldn't be treating him? There wasn't much that got us both upset, but this really tested us.

I told Jerry I'd go down and pick up his records. Still a car salesperson, I had a variable schedule. He'd already missed work for the doctor appointments and tests, and this was one thing I could do so that he didn't need to miss another half day. I called Dr. Lance's staff to inform them I was coming to the doctor's office the next day to pick up copies of Jerry's records.

When I arrived, the receptionist and nursing staff were less than cooperative. I had driven more than an hour, and I grew a bit testy as they continued to allege they weren't Jerry's records, but theirs.

I contended that Jerry's records were pertinent only to him, and without a patient to treat, the records had no value to them whatsoever.

The verbal jousting continued until I'd been pushed to my limit.

Finally, speaking loudly, so that all three patients in the waiting room could hear, I said, "I will make a scene, here in your office, in front of your patients, and I will come back every day to do the same until you hand over my husband's records. Those documents won't do you any good at all since we have *zero* confidence in the doctor's ability to treat my husband."

They finally acquiesced, and I walked out of the office with Jerry's records in hand.

We really shouldn't have needed to have that altercation. The office staff had tried to intimidate us, and while medical records may technically belong to the doctor's office, our data is *our* data. We are entitled to copies of our own medical records.

I include this to help you understand that, quite often, when we buck the system, issues arise. It's critical to take courage, understand your rights, and stand up for what you want and believe. After all, it is *your* body and *your* health, and each of us needs to take charge of doing what is best for our well-being. Sometimes we need an advocate to help us stay strong with our decisions, but oftentimes we can and must rise up to be our own advocate.

As I walked out of the building and toward my car, with his medical records in hand, I realized Jerry and I had taken an important step—away from blindly doing everything the doctors said, and toward becoming actively involved in our own health care decisions.

□

Two days after our appointment with the new oncologist, Jerry returned to Dr. PM's medical office and dropped off his records. We wanted to make sure Dr. PM had adequate time to review and share them with his associates before Jerry's next appointment.

A week after our first appointment with Dr. PM, after he had reviewed Jerry's medical records, we returned to Dr. PM's intriguingly eclectic office.

After exchanging pleasantries, he opened Jerry's file. "My colleagues and I have had an opportunity to review the test results and interpretations of the CT and PET scans, and the biopsy. We deliberated over the conflicting diagnoses and test results, and concur, for several reasons, that the cancer in your lymph node is lung cancer, not testicular cancer. Usually, a recurrence of lung cancer happens four to six months after the initial cancer appears, not four years later. The fact that it has taken so long to surface is the good news."

Why, when it came to oncology, did the doctors always seem to have good news and bad news?

Dr. PM continued. "However, a recurrence of lung cancer is usually very aggressive. With the lung cancer now appearing outside the lung, we have to categorize it as stage IIIB."

I felt dread sinking in my gut, and I didn't even know what stage IIIB was.

"Typically, stage IIIB lung cancer gives you about four to six months."

Four to six months. The doctor just gave my Jerry a death sentence.

☐

The only way I can share the oncologist's prognosis with you is because, while researching our records to write this chapter, I came across it in the doctor's notes. The facts are there, in print.

The reality is that I have wrestled countless times over the words in Dr. PM's notes, trying to recall anything that would jar my memory of that day and time period. Slowly, very slowly and painfully, I am remembering fragments of the visit. I sit, and ponder, and pray, and try to breathe. I have this ache where my heart should be. I want to be able to remember more.

I can still visualize the exam rooms and the chemo room, the station where they'd take Jerry's blood pressure, and the scale to check his weight. I see the receptionist's desk, and the waiting area with all the sickly patients and their support people—family, friends, or caregivers.

But to this day, I have no recollection of Dr. PM uttering those devastating words. I expect I buried the memory of the prognosis, along with repressing many events that took place around this cancer. Some nontraumatic memories and situations stand out, and I remember them clearly, like the appearance of the waiting area. On the whole, however, I still struggle to recall many of the memories during this time.

With frustration, I also think back to the question I'd asked Dr. Blinders, Jerry's first oncologist. "Since Jerry has been diagnosed with cancer, should he give up smoking cigarettes?" Dr. Blinders had said, "No, giving it up would be too stressful." Then Jerry had been diagnosed with lung cancer. Four years after the cancerous part of his lung had been removed, Jerry was diagnosed with terminal lung cancer.

Even now, my mind reels. *Giving up smoking sooner would have been more stressful than this?*

☐

Dr. PM's prescribed treatment for Jerry's lymph node cancer called for six cycles of chemotherapy comprised of a Taxol and carboplatin cocktail, followed by three cycles of Taxotere. Additionally, he would receive six weeks of radiation.

As before, we were set on the hamster wheel of treatment.

Jerry, my flannel man, was a trooper. After the first few treatments, he often drove the hour-plus to his chemo/radiation appointments and then on to work. Each time, I offered to go with him, or drive, but after I'd attended his first few sessions and everything had gone well, he assured me it wasn't necessary.

Jerry, an avid reader, frequently had a book in hand. He would fill the hours of receiving chemo infusions by reading, visiting with other chemo recipients, or napping.

On rare occasions, when he wanted me to go with him to the oncologist or a chemo/radiation appointment, I took a few hours off from my job at the car dealership and went.

We tried to live our lives as normally and routinely as possible, not giving in to the cancer or letting it rule our lives. We'd always been people who just made up our minds and then got things done, whether Jerry had cancer or not. And that was what we continued to do.

Sometime during Jerry's treatment, I found an article that piqued my curiosity. I'd developed an interest in nutritional supplements and natural health products years prior, after finding one that had helped me tremendously with a badly broken ankle. I came to understand that our bodies have the amazing ability to heal themselves if we give them what they need.

We could compare the human body to a computer. We've all heard the phrase *garbage in, garbage out*, yes? If the data we enter into the computer isn't any good, the results won't be good either. Likewise, if we eat highly processed fast food, junk food, or nutritionally deficient food, how can our bodies perform optimally?

We need to stop giving our bodies things that make them sick and start giving them things that help them heal.

I'd subscribed to *Alternatives*, the intriguing newsletter of Dr. David Williams, a chiropractor, biochemist, and medical researcher who'd developed a reputation as one of the world's leading authorities on natural healing. His exclusive natural treatments and remedies, often uncovered in far-flung places such as the African bush or Australian Outback, are usually years ahead of those offered by conventional medicine. Dr. Williams' mission is to provide those committed to good health the best resources available to support the body's innate ability to heal itself.

I enjoyed Dr. William's newsletters. First and foremost, he focused on educating and challenging his readers and the medical community. He wasn't writing hype to promote the latest product he was selling, the way we often see products marketed today. Instead he sold subscriptions to his newsletter to provide his readers with sound and proven alternatives to conventional medicine and medical protocols.

In one issue of his newsletter, I found an article about AHCC (active hexose correlated compound), an extract derived from certain mushrooms that are considered medicinal in many parts of the world.

Here are a few quotes from his 2005 article "The Easiest Way to Cheat Cancer Ever." (My emphases are in *italics*.)

> Cancer cells are naturally present in everyone's bloodstream, but are kept in check by special immune cells called NK (short for "natural killer").

> In Japan . . . the most successful cancer treatment involves stimulating the patient's immune system so tumors are gobbled up in a feeding frenzy of NK cells. . . . *Strengthening the human immune system holds the best promise of finding tomorrow's real cures.*

> Medical studies indicate this (AHCC) may be the most powerful human immune booster ever tested. Studies show that taking the capsules *increases NK cell activity by 300 percent or more*! Even NASA is impressed. They now use this Japanese immune-booster to prevent and treat infections in astronauts.

> *And unlike many cancer treatments that weaken the patient over time, this new treatment makes patients healthier and stronger by increasing the immune function. . . . It greatly improves survival rates, while reducing the bad side effects of chemo and radiation.*

I shared the article with Jerry. Although he tended to be skeptical of natural healing, the mention of NASA and reducing the bad effects of chemo and radiation appealed to him. We both found the information compelling enough to bring the article to the attention of the oncologist.

Dr. PM didn't say that Jerry couldn't take the supplement, but he became cynical and mocked us for considering something outside of conventional medicine. His attitude was condescending, like patting a child on the head and saying, "There, there. You can if it will make you feel better."

We felt extremely disappointed in the doctor's response, but also hopeful about what we'd read in the report, since, as opposed to injecting sick patients with poison, this actually made sense. "Strengthening the human immune system holds the best promise of finding tomorrow's real cures." To Jerry and me, it was worth a try.

Jerry incorporated AHCC into his daily routine. Although he'd always disliked taking pills, and often gagged while swallowing them, Jerry took AHCC faithfully every day.

We hoped, and waited, to see how they would affect his cancer.

☐

This chemo didn't have as many side effects as with his first cancer. I'm not sure if the reason was a new anti-nausea medication, the different chemo, smaller dosages, or the AHCC mushroom extract, or a combination, but Jerry didn't have as much nausea, and it wasn't nearly as intense, as before. He also didn't lose his hair, which delighted him, but he did experience neuropathy— numbness in his hands and feet.

If you recall, he had experienced some chemo induced peripheral neuropathy (CIPN) during his first cancer treatment, coupled with circulation issues, which had primarily affected his left leg. This neuropathy was different, affecting both his feet and his hands. The pain, burning, tingling, and loss of feeling grew particularly bothersome in his hands.

Like many couples, Jerry and I could never agree on temperatures. I always felt cold, and he always felt hot. Early in our marriage I'd learned to wear layers, and for thirty years had even kept a lap blanket to cover up with in the car while he ran the air-conditioning. I didn't say anything, just covered up. He'd often look at me and ask, "You're *cold*?" in utter disbelief.

One side effect from the chemo that affected Jerry during this third cancer treatment was that he often felt incredibly cold, even colder than me. Somehow,

I don't think I was very sympathetic. Whenever he mentioned how cold he was, I largely heard it as whining and complaining, and thought, *What goes around, comes around.* I'd tell him to put on a sweatshirt, jacket, or jeans instead of shorts.

While he felt cold, I experienced the opposite temperature challenge—hot flashes. I chuckle as I recall that, in the entire history of our marriage, it was the only time we could somewhat agree on where to set the thermostat.

☐

Though Jerry didn't experience as many side effects from the chemo, the radiation was far more devastating. Technology had improved to target smaller areas with less impact on surrounding tissues. However, it was impossible to radiate the nodule in his neck without impacting Jerry's esophagus.

To say he had a sore throat would be an understatement. He had a lot of pain and difficulty just swallowing. The radiation left Jerry's throat so inflamed that at times he couldn't eat, drink, or even swallow his own spit.

The oncologist asked questions about Jerry's esophageal symptoms, pain, and severity. Then, to our disappointment, he merely told Jerry to eat small, frequent meals.

There were entire days when Jerry could barely swallow at all!

Dr. PM wrote out a prescription that was supposed to help. Then he sent Jerry to his next radiation appointment.

☐

Earlier I shared with you that my heart aches each time I learn that someone is diagnosed with cancer, because I have a good idea of the journey ahead of them. *So* many side effects accompany conventional cancer treatments. Everyone who undergoes chemo, radiation, or surgery has stories to tell. Some share them while others suffer in silence. For those who've never been in the military and served during war or conflict, their cancer experience may be the most horrific event of their lives.

We often become focused on and consumed with our own terrible ordeals, and yet if we try to gain perspective in considering others' battles, we may find compassion for and connection with them, and find calming in our own journey.

All of us, cancer patients and their families, like soldiers and first responders and their families, undergo extreme traumas, and must heal from the horrors inflicted and encounters endured.

If you must experience and recover from hell on Earth, it's best to do it with positive and helpful family and friends. Thankfully Jerry and I were blessed with uplifting support, but most of all, what got us through day to day was each other.

☐

One afternoon I walked into Jerry's office at home while he typed away at his computer. He'd just been down to the kitchen trying to find something he could eat or drink. I knew it wasn't a good time to ask what he wanted me to make for dinner, because his throat hurt from the radiation.

It was so hard. He wanted to eat but couldn't. Cold drinks didn't help. Neither did warm. His throat was so swollen and inflamed he could barely swallow a drop of water. He was frustrated, hungry, and in pain.

But I wanted to take care of him, and in my world at the time, food was love, and love was food. I set my hands on his shoulders and rested my chin on the top of his head. "What can I get you for dinner?" I asked.

He sat back in his chair, lightly leaning into me. "Nothing. It hurts too much to eat."

Silence followed as I tried to think what he might be able to have that could soothe his throat or go down easily. I knew better than to start listing off choices that would only frustrate him further.

"Diane, I know you'd run to the store to get me anything I thought I could eat or drink, but there isn't anything I even want to try."

He shifted away from me and seemed to study the computer screen. His voice, emotionless, said, "You know, if it's my time, it's my time. God's will be done."

His words sucked the wind out of me, then hit me like a truck.

I struggled to process them, not knowing how to respond.

The words echoed in my mind. *If it's my time . . . God's will be done.* On a certain level, I think I understood. He'd made his peace with God. I really didn't believe he was giving up. He was simply assuring me that he was secure in his faith.

But I wasn't ready to hear it! Everything that was strong in me drained out, and numbness set in. I had nothing to say in response.

It would take a bit for me to recuperate from those words. I think it was the first time in Jerry's three cancer battles that either one of us had mentioned his mortality.

The cumulative effect of radiation and chemotherapy took a serious toll on Jerry. The chills, as well as neuropathy in his hands and feet, were becoming intolerable.

He also experienced soreness and weakening in his shoulder from the radiation. It made wearing a seat belt unbearable, so Jerry had to move the shoulder strap behind his back when driving or riding in the car.

A few weeks after he finished his radiation, Jerry developed a fever and shortness of breath. He called Dr. PM to let him know. The doctor prescribed antibiotics, but after a week they still hadn't helped.

Jerry went to his August oncology appointment in misery. The doctor sent Jerry straight to the ER, and the hospital admitted him with radiation pneumonia.

He spent one night in the hospital. They got the fever down, and he returned home.

Our next appointment with Dr. PM a few days later felt solemn. Like so many people I've known who have endured chemotherapy, it seemed the doctors take them to the edge of what the body can handle, and then the patient has to stop chemo treatments before completing the doctor's prescribed dosage.

I couldn't begin to guess how many I've talked to who said that they, or their mom, dad, sibling, or friend hadn't finished the course of treatment because their body just couldn't take it anymore.

Dr. PM admitted, "Jerry, you shouldn't have any more chemo. The impact and ramifications of more chemo would be too hard on you in the long run."

Jerry considered that. "If I cut the final treatment, then the cancer might return. I'll go through the last chemo treatment. I want to make certain the cancer doesn't come back."

The doctor said, "Jerry, it would be detrimental to your health to have the last treatment."

I agreed.

Soon after, Jerry conceded.

We left Dr. PM's office, Jerry now finished with his treatment for cancer three and on the road to healing from the chemo and radiation side effects.

For his third cancer, Jerry had received fourteen doses of chemo. Adding that to his original forty-six doses for his first cancer, he'd now undergone sixty doses of chemotherapy.

About three months after Dr. PM discontinued Jerry's chemo, Jerry went in for a CT of the chest, abdomen, and pelvis. No cancer was found, nor was anything else to be concerned about.

Jerry dutifully followed up with his oncologist every three months, then every six months for years. Cancer three did not return.

☐

I always ordered four-month supplies of AHCC mushroom extract. Each time Jerry got down to the last bottle, he said, "I'm on my last bottle of AHCC. You need to order more."

It makes me chuckle to think that Jerry entrusted me to take care of this aspect of his life when he did pretty much everything else himself. I don't know why, but it amuses me.

Chemo and radiation had killed the lung cancer that had appeared in his lymph node, according to the oncologist, and so Jerry was in remission. When Jerry went in for his checkups, the doctor occasionally mocked him, asking if he was still taking his "psychedelic mushrooms." Thus, the name "Dr. PM."

Jerry always replied that he was.

They were not psychedelic, but medicinal. Mushrooms have been proven to have *many* healing properties. Personally, I took offense at the doctor's attitude, but Jerry had a better relationship with him and let the comments slide.

Did the AHCC help? We can't say that, but Jerry blew past the four to six-month sentence he'd been given, and it was six years before cancer surfaced again.

Chapter 6
Spring 2017—The Quest for Truth:
Cancer Three

I sat at the kitchen table sipping a hot cup of tea. The stack of medical records for Jerry's third cancer lay before me. Was it worth my time and energy? After all, what were the chances that I'd even find anything else out of the ordinary? We'd moved to a different state, from Texas to Illinois, so we hadn't gone to the same oncologist as with cancers one and two.

As I reflected on how Jerry's third cancer had played out, I thought of the two Illinois doctors he'd gone to. They'd been opposites. We had changed oncologists because we'd had no confidence in Dr. Lance, while Dr. PM had portrayed professionalism and assurance. However, that image had become tarnished over the course of treatment, at least in my mind, when his attitude had grown condescending and a bit arrogant.

As with the documents for cancers one and two, I wasn't sure what I was looking for. I just sat there, lost in thought, my mind settling on nothing.

All at once the words and vision returned: *Sifting. Contrast. Light/dark. Truth/lies. Good/evil.* A wire mesh in motion. Nuggets of gravel falling into the mesh and collecting. Sand being sifted through.

Somehow, those opposites had to do with why God was having me write such a different book than the one I'd planned.

I took a deep breath, grabbed the "Dr. Lance" stack, the first Illinois oncologist, and opened the top file.

These records started in 2003, shortly after we'd moved to Illinois. I really didn't expect to find anything from 2003 to 2005, the two years between cancers two and three, but I thought it best to review it all. Leafing through Jerry's medical history, the doctor's notes, and routine CT scans, I thought, *Yep, not much here.*

As I started reading Dr. Lance's notes from March 18, 2005, the beginning of Jerry's third cancer, there were no surprises. Dr. Lance had incorporated the results of the CT scan and ordered a PET scan. Jerry had developed a mass in his right neck/collarbone area, just as I remembered the diagnosis.

And then I read this.

	Hospital		Attending Dr :	
, IL.			Admitting Dr :	
			Consulting Dr :	

I M A G I N G

Procedure:	Procedure Date/Time:	Accession #:
CT PELVIS W CON	3/18/05 7:34:05 PM	CT
CT CHEST W CON	3/18/05 7:34:02 PM	CT
CT ABDOMEN WO/W CON	3/18/05 7:32:35 PM	CT

CPT 4

72193, 72193, 71260, 71260, 74170, 74170, 0

CT OF THE CHEST, ABDOMEN AND PELVIS

HISTORY OF ADENOPATHY.

TECHNIQUE: Axial images were obtained from the lung apices through the pelvis following the administration of oral and IV contrast. Precontrast exam was obtained of the liver.

Comparison is made to the prior study of December 15, 2003. Reference of prior study of June 30, 2003.

There is pleural thickening in the apices bilaterally which remains unchanged. There is a focal area of irregular linear densities in the right upper lobe which are compatible with scarring. This is unchanged from the prior exam, as well as from the previous study. There is also irregular linear densities in the subpleural region along the right hemithorax in the lower lung, again suggesting scarring. This remains unchanged. There is no pleural effusion or evidence of consolidation. No masses are identified. There remains elevation of the right hemidiaphragm which is unchanged from the previous study.

The cardiac size is normal and no pericardial effusion is present. The great vessels appear within normal limits. There is no mediastinal, hilar or axillary adenopathy. There is a small subcentimeter node in the subcarinal region which is unchanged from the previous study. There is a 3 x 3 cm irregular soft tissue mass in the lower cervical triangle or medial supraclavicular region on the right, new from the prior exam. This is likely matted nodes.

There is diffuse decreased density of the liver compatible with a fatty infiltration. This is unchanged from the prior exam. The spleen is normal in size without focal masses. There is an adjacent small accessory spleen. Adrenals are normal. Gallbladder and pancreas are within normal limits. The kidneys show normal contrast uptake and excretion bilaterally. The ureters show normal course and caliber. Urinary bladder is normally distended. There remains mild thickening of the wall of the urinary bladder. This was present on prior study and not appreciably changed allowing for the difference in distention. There is no inguinal or pelvic adenopathy noted. The aorta is normal in caliber. There is a soft tissue mass between the aorta and vena cava

Send To:		Pt Name : HUSSEY, JERRY	Sex : MALE
		Pt Phone :	Age : 55 Years
		Ord Dr :	Svc
		MR #	Req Loc :
. .		DOB :	Pt Loc :
		Billing # :	

March 18, 2005, document

The size of the mass had been 3 x 3 cm. I knew Jerry had had a mass in the neck area, but I didn't remember that it had been 3 cm.

I resumed reading. "This is likely matted nodes." So, what does that mean? I opened my laptop and accessed the Internet. (My clarification is in parentheses.)

> Typically, when lymph nodes are referred to as "matted" it means that upon palpation (feeling/pushing), the nodes appear to move in a connected fashion. Nodes that are matted can be either benign or malignant, but in malignant cases, "matted nodes" typically is a warning sign of a poor prognosis.[13]

---

[13] http://www.answers.com/Q/What_are_matted_lymph_nodes

Facetiously, I muttered, "Well that doesn't sound too good." Often I'm a master of understatement, and by minimizing what I'd just read, it gave me the opportunity to process and try to reduce the sting. Although I knew how the rest of cancer three had played out, reading the words "warning sign of a poor prognosis" haunted me.

Based on that report, Dr. Lance had ordered a PET scan, which had confirmed it was cancer.

My fingers curled into my hair. This mass in Jerry's neck had been the same size as the mass that Dr. Blinders had ignored in Jerry's lung four and a half years prior—3 cm. Ironic that the two cancers had been the same size. Thankfully, this time, the doctor hadn't chosen to ignore the mass, though he hadn't been able to determine whether it was metastasized testicular or lung cancer. I released my hair.

My next step was to examine the results of the PET scan.

Within moments I was speechless. The history was almost entirely inaccurate. History: "underwent right orchiectomy (testicle removed) 6/2001 for germ cell seminoma. This was followed by adjuvant chemotherapy."

Yes, the testicle was removed 6/2/2001, but Jerry had received chemotherapy before, not after!

"He also was noted to have right upper lobe malignancy treated with chemotherapy for non-small cell carcinoma."

No, he was not! He was never treated for his first lung cancer with chemotherapy! Two cancers, one chemotherapy, not two and two. Also, the history shows no mention of the surgery to remove the right upper lobe of Jerry's lung!

I understand that mistakes can be made in summarizing and transcription, but three key points in this history are wrong or excluded! Jerry would never have given that account of his history to anyone. Was it a clerical error? Or was Dr. Lance guilty of not really listening to Jerry? He'd had copies of all Jerry's records from San Antonio. Had he ever bothered to read them?

Was the error made by the office doing the PET scan? Or Dr. Lance's office? Where did they get this history?

Everyone involved in a patient's care relies on the information written in the medical records—doctors, nurses, and technicians, and others. When the information is wrong, it can lead to other errors, potentially life-threatening! I shook my head at the incompetency.

Moving on in the report, the 3/22/2005 PET scan showed the metastatic nodule to be either 26 or 25 mm (a mistake within the report itself; whichever size is a slight variation from the 3 cm or 30 mm result from the CT scan).

Now, either that's sloppy paperwork, or the mass shrank while someone was typing the report. Grr! So many mistakes in one document!

(I would come to find many more errors in Jerry's medical records. I encourage everyone to ask for a copy of their medical records to ensure accuracy and accountability.)

Telling myself to simmer down, I went online again to find the definition of a couple of terms from the report:

- **NSCLC:** non-small cell lung cancer
- **SUV (Standardized Uptake Value):** This basically shows how brightly the nodule shows up on the PET scan. The brightness is directly correlated to the ferocity of the cancer in feeding on the sugar. "An SUV of 2.5 or higher is generally considered to be indicative of malignant tissue."[14] And Jerry had been at 4.8.

Following is the entire document.

---

[14] https://www.sciencedirect.com/topics/medicine-and-dentistry/standardized-uptake-value

```
Medical Imaging          PATIENT NAME:    HUSSEY, JERRY

              , IL           DATE OF BIRTH:
866-                         PATIENT ID:
                             ACCOUNT NUMBER:
                             EXAM DATE:       03/22/05

         Medical Imaging     REF PHYSICIAN:   DR.


DR.

              , IL
```

PET WHOLE BODY IMAGING SCAN

HISTORY:	PET imaging for restaging NSCLC. This is a 55 year old man who underwent right orchiectomy 6/2001 for germ cell seminoma. This was followed by adjuvant chemotherapy. He also was noted to have right upper lobe malignancy treated with chemotherapy for non-small cell carcinoma.
TECHNIQUE:	14.1 mCi of FDG were injected with fasting blood sugar of 93 followed by PET whole body imaging and CT for co-registration.

FINDINGS:

NECK/CHEST:
Metabolic FDG images were co-registered with axial CT. There is hypermetabolic 26 mm metastatic nodal aggregate in the right supraclavicular region with SUV of 4.8. This is likely related to known right upper lobe NSCLC. There is no recurrent hypermetabolic tumor within the right lung. There is no evidence of hilar or mediastinal metastatic disease.

ABDOMEN/PELVIS:
Metabolic FDG images were co-registered with axial CT. There is normal physiologic metabolic low-level tissue background activity present with no evidence of primary or metastatic malignancy. Specifically, there is no evidence of recurrent retroperitoneal nodal metastatic disease.

SKELETON:
There is normal low-level skeletal activity present with no evidence of bony metastatic disease.

IMPRESSION:
Hypermetabolic 25 mm right supraclavicular metastatic nodal aggregate likely from known lung primary.

```
                    , MD
LM:          : 3/22/05
        Thank you for referring this patient to          Medical Imaging
```

March 22, 2005, document

I continued reading, until my gaze stuck on this phrase.

IMPRESSION:
Hypermetabolic 25 mm right supraclavicular metastatic nodal aggregate likely from known lung primary.

from March 22, 2005, document

Jerry's second cancer had been non-small cell lung cancer, and this third cancer was *likely* related to that? It was there in black and white . . . but Dr. Lance had told us that they couldn't determine what type of cancer Jerry had, saying it might be either lung or testicular. He had been eager to refer us to Lance Armstrong's doctors—testicular cancer specialists—but the PET scan report indicated *likely* lung cancer.

My simmering thoughts approached boiling point.

Slow down, Diane. You haven't gone through everything yet. I strived for a measure of objectivity, with limited success, and continued reading.

Jerry's next appointment with Dr. Lance had been on March 24, two days after the PET scan. These were Dr. Lance's own notes about the visit:

Oncology and Hematology,

PATIENT: Hussey, Jerry	**DATE SEEN:** <u>03/24/2005</u>
ACCOUNT#:	**OFFICE:**

FOLLOW-UP VISIT

SUBJECTIVE:
Mr. Hussey is a 55-year-old

He has a history of two primary malignancies, the first being a testicular cancer and the second being a non-small cell lung cancer diagnosed approximately four years ago. The patient is here to see me today because of a new swelling of his right lower neck. He was found to have a palpable right supraclavicular lymph node. In fact, recent CT scan performed at _____ on March 18 did confirm a new 3-cm mass in the right supraclavicular lower circle triangle region. Because of this I ordered a whole body imaging scan, which did show a hypermetabolic 25-mm right supraclavicular metastatic nodule felt to be lung primary. In addition, I did order tumor markers for his testicular cancer including LDH, alpha-fetoprotein, and beta-hCG, which were all within normal limits. The rest of his blood work, including liver function tests, is within normal limits as well.

REVIEW OF SYSTEMS:
GENERAL: No fevers, chills or night sweats.
HEENT: No headache, blurry vision or diplopia. No mouth pain.
RESPIRATORY: No cough or shortness of breath.
CARDIOVASCULAR: No chest pain.
GI: No abdominal pain, nausea, vomiting, diarrhea or constipation. No melena or hematochezia.
GU: No hematuria or dysuria.
NEURO: No weakness. No paresthesias.
MUSCULOSKELETAL: No bone pain.

PHYSICAL EXAMINATION:
GENERAL: The patient is alert and oriented x three and in no apparent distress.
VITAL SIGNS: Blood pressure 160/98, pulse 88, temperature 96.8, respirations 18, weight 226.

ASSESSMENT:
1. New 3-cm right supraclavicular lymph node.
2. History of poorly differentiated non-small cell lung cancer, status post right upper lobe lobectomy.

March 24, 2005, document

Odd, to say the least. ". . . Imaging scan, which did show a . . . nodule felt to be a lung primary. In addition, I did order tumor markers for his testicular cancer . . . which were all within normal limits."

Yes, I supposed it made sense to rule out metastasized testicular cancer by ordering tumor markers, but the nodule was "felt to be a lung primary." Why hadn't Dr. Lance ordered testing to confirm or exclude lung cancer as well?

Like a detective, I found myself questioning everything. At the time, my husband's life had been in this man's hands.

I moved on to the next document, the first page of Jerry's biopsy.

Hospital
Department of Pathology

Surgical Pathology Report

Location: OUTPATIENT-H
Med. Rec. #:
Billing #:
Birth Date/Age/Sex: (Age: 55) M

Specimen #:
Patient: HUSSEY, JERRY
Physician:

Date Specimen Collected: 3/31/2005
Date Specimen Received: 3/31/2005
Date & Time Reported: 4/1/2005 15:41

Clinical Information:
RIGHT SUPRACLAVICULAR NODE; ADENOCARCINOMA, LUNG; TESTICULAR GERMINOMA

Specimen(s) Submitted:
A. Supraclavicular node core biopsy under CT guided, right

Final Pathologic Diagnosis:

A. Right supraclavicular node CT guided core biopsy:
    Metastatic poorly differentiated adenocarcinoma with focal necrosis, consistent with
    the clinical history of embryonal carcinoma of the testes.

em   , M.D.
                                              ** Electronic Signature (   ) **
Addendum:

Addendum Diagnosis:
Immunostaining for Cytokeratin 20, which is a marker for colonic carcinoma, is negative in tumor cells.
Immunostaining for Cytokeratin 7, which is a marker for carcinoma other than colonic, is strongly positive in
tumor cells.
Immunostaining for TTF-1, which is a marker for lung adenocarcinoma, is positive in a low percentage of the
nuclei.
Immunostaining for Beta HCG, which is a marker for germ cell tumors, is positive in many of the tumor cells.
Immunostaining for Cytokeratin AE1/3 is strongly positive in tumor cells.
Immunostaining for Alpha-fetoprotein, which is a marker for germ cell tumors, is negative in tumor cells.
The finding are non-conclusive by the presence of very few positive nuclei for TTF-1 and mostly positive
cytoplasmic staining for HCG as well as strong positive staining for cytokeratin made me favor germ cell tumor
as the primary site in this case, but adenocarcinoma of the lung cannot be totally excluded.

                                              **Electronic Signature (   ) **
                                              4/11/2005

Page 1   Continued on Next Page
                          Hospital   Barrington, IL
                          Office: Fax:

March 31, 2005, document (page 1 of 2)

My brain felt twisted like a pretzel. It wasn't enough to read the test results. I'd have to *understand* what the report said, which meant a lot of online research and note-taking. The process left me drained.

This biopsy report got set aside multiple times. Did I really need to delve into all the details? Ultimately, yes, but it would take time to clear my head, and pick it up with rested eyes and fresh resolve.

After a prolonged rest, the clear mind and fresh resolve were ready to go.

"TTF-1, which is a marker for lung adenocarcinoma, is positive."

"Beta HCG, which is a marker for germ cell (testicular) tumors, is positive."

"Alpha-fetoprotein, which is a marker for germ cell (testicular) tumors, is negative."

"The finding (sic) are non-conclusive."

I turned to page 2.

March 31, 2005, document (page 2 of 2)

Thomas Ulbright . . . on University Boulevard in Indianapolis. I went online. Thomas Ulbright was a well-known oncologist. He had been part of Lance Armstrong's cancer team.

Seeing that hand-written note tied my stomach in knots. It almost seemed that Dr. Lance, our first Illinois oncologist, had wanted to get connected to Lance Armstrong's team of doctors through Jerry. I recalled what he'd said in his office at our last meeting.

"So, you have three options. One, you can treat it as lung cancer. Two, treat it as testicular cancer, through me. Or three, you can treat it as testicular cancer through Lance Armstrong's doctors."

Throughout this spring of 2017, there were times I'd sit and ponder what I was reading. I'd often spend hours researching, processing, and trying to understand each element I uncovered. But on occasion, I'd be so enraged at the discoveries that I'd have to walk away from it and try to deal with the emotions. This was one of those reports.

When I finally came back with my objectivity intact, I allowed for the possibility that Dr. Lance had simply been doing his homework before we'd arrived at Jerry's last appointment with him. He had been fully prepared to connect us with Lance Armstrong's doctors.

Our last meeting with Dr. Lance had been April 8, so I pulled out his notes from that appointment. Dr. Lance had written the following within one to two days after Jerry and I had walked out. It further raised my eyebrows, and then my hackles.

I never would have seen this if I hadn't gone back and gotten Jerry's records to give to Dr. PM.

PATIENT: Hussey, Jerry   **DATE SEEN:** <u>04/08/2005</u>

ACCOUNT#: [ ]   **OFFICE:** [ ]

FOLLOW-UP VISIT

SUBJECTIVE:
Mr. Hussey is a 55-year-old white male with past medical history significant for a large retroperitoneal seminoma treated with carboplatin and etoposide approximately four years ago. In addition, he has a history of a poorly differentiated nonsmall cell lung cancer status post right upper lobe lobectomy. I initially started seeing Jerry because of a new 3-cm right supraclavicular lymph node. CAT scan showed increased activity. I send him for a CT-guided biopsy which came back consistent with a metastatic poorly differentiated adenocarcinoma with focal necrosis. On the past report, it was mentioned that it was consistent with the clinical history of an embryonal carcinoma of the testes. After discussion with Dr.   , I did inform him that this patient also had an adenocarcinoma of the lung. Because of this, he is going to stain the tissue for further diagnostic purposes. With the exception of feeling somewhat anxious, Jerry has no significant complaints.

REVIEW OF SYSTEMS:
GENERAL: No fevers, chills or night sweats.
HEENT: No headache, blurry vision or diplopia. No mouth pain.
RESPIRATORY: He does have a nonproductive cough.
CARDIOVASCULAR: No chest pain.
GI: No abdominal pain, nausea, vomiting, diarrhea or constipation. No melena or hematochezia.
GU: No hematuria or dysuria.
NEURO: No weakness. No paresthesias.
MUSCULOSKELETAL: No bone pain.

PHYSICAL EXAMINATION:
GENERAL: The patient is alert and oriented times three in no apparent distress.
VITAL SIGNS: Blood pressure 136/80, pulse 80, temperature 97.4, respiratory rate is 18. Weight is 218 pounds.

ASSESSMENT:
1. Probable metastatic poorly differentiated adenocarcinoma.
2. History of poorly differentiated nonsmall cell lung cancer status post right upper lobe lobectomy.
3. History of retroperitoneal seminoma status post chemotherapy.

PLAN:
The patient's tumor will be restained for further differentiation. He will come back and see me on Thursday for follow-up visit. I will call him with the results once I have an answer.

4/13/2005

April 8, 2005, document

"On the past report it was mentioned that [the adenocarcinoma] was consistent with the clinical history of an embryonal carcinoma of the testes. After discussion with Dr. ___ (the pathologist), I did inform him that this patient also had an adenocarcinoma of the lung."

"After discussion" apparently meant a new discussion. Hadn't Dr. Lance emphasized both of Jerry's previous cancers to the pathologist, at the outset?

"Because of this, he (the pathologist) is going to stain the tissue for further diagnostic purposes." Why weren't both the potential testicular and lung cancers given equal attention before this point?

> IMPRESSION:
> Hypermetabolic 25 mm right supraclavicular metastatic nodal aggregate likely from known lung primary.

from March 22, 2005, document

". . . Likely from known lung primary" had been the stated impression from the beginning. Why had Dr. Lance dismissed that?

> nodule felt to be lung primary. In addition, I did order tumor markers for his testicular cancer including LDH, alpha-fetoprotein, and beta-hCG, which were all within normal limits.

from March 24, 2005, document

"I did order tumor markers for his testicular cancer."

Did the fault lay with the pathologist, or with Dr. Lance and a professional interest in connecting with Thomas Ulbright on University Boulevard in Indianapolis?

Or, had Dr. Lance simply been incompetent?

During our last visit, he hadn't mentioned to us that he was going to order the tissue stained "for further diagnostic purposes." Had the "further diagnostic purposes" been a way to cover his backside?

> PLAN:
> The patient's tumor will be restained for further differentiation. He will come back and see me on Thursday for follow-up visit. I will call him with the results once I have an answer.

from April 8, 2005, document

"The patient's tumor will be re-stained for further differentiation," he'd decided after we'd walked out of his office.

I looked at it from every angle and couldn't come up with any other explanations that connected all the pieces of why testicular cancer had become the focus instead of lung cancer. It made me feel physically ill, and I was disgusted with Dr. Lance.

Whether incompetent or career motivated, he could have harmed Jerry, had we not gone to a different doctor. Will I ever be able to put into words what that does to me?

Setting Dr. Lance's paperwork aside, I realized that almost all of cancer three still lay before me, in the pile of Illinois oncologist two, Dr. PM's, documents.

But Dr. PM had been far more professional, so undoubtedly this was (finally) going to get easier.

As a parting thought before I close out this chapter, *please* remember that you are entitled to copies of your own medical records! It is your body and your health. After each appointment, ask for copies or access them online. And then read them!

Chapter 7
Spring 2017—The Quest for Truth:
Cancer Three, Continued

Diving now into Dr. PM's records, I wondered, How *had* Dr. PM and his twelve colleagues swiftly determined Jerry's third cancer had been metastasized lung cancer?

I glanced through Dr. PM's consultation notes from our first visit on April 19, 2005.

> supraclavicular lymph node. Core biopsy demonstrates metastatic carcinoma. Special stains reveal a positive TTF-1 and also a positive beta-HCG. Cytokeratin stains are also positive. There is apparently a discrep ancy between the pathology interpretation, which suggests a recurrent germ cell tumor, and his oncologist who believes this is more likely recurrent lung carcinoma. He is

from April 19, 2005, document (page 1)

"There is apparently a discrepancy between the pathology interpretation, which suggests a recurrent germ cell tumor, and his oncologist who believes this is more likely a recurrent lung carcinoma." What? When had Dr. Lance changed his mind? That was the opposite impression Jerry and I had been left with as we'd walked out of Dr. Lance's office the last time.

I shook my head as I tried to comprehend the about-face. I could only surmise that Dr. Lance had attempted to cover himself: "After discussion with Dr. ___ (the pathologist), I did inform him that this patient also had an adenocarcinoma of the lung. . . . The patient's tumor will be re-stained for further differentiation."

On the next page, another note of Dr. PM caught my attention, under "Impression."

DATA REVIEW: Biopsies are reviewed with Dr.   in the Pathology Department and are as described above. Dr.   's impression is that this represents a non-small cell lung carcinoma.

IMPRESSION: Metastatic carcinoma right supraclavicular fossa , likely metastatic non-small cell lung carcinoma. The pathologic features do not support a metastatic germ cell tumor. However, the slides are to reviewed in the pathology QA process. TTF-1 is a fairly specific lung cancer marker and B-HCG is well described in NSCCL. We would not expect this degree of B-HCG in a seminoma.

PLAN:
Mr.Hussey will obtain his prior treatme nt records from his testicular tumor and his current scans for my review prior to any definitive treatment planning. The pathology interpretation certainly suggests a recurrence of his lung carcinoma rather than his testicular carcinoma. Since treatment and prognosis are quite divergent with these potential diagnoses, efforts to be as certain as possible about the nature of th is process will be explored. He is to return after I can review his entire records.

CC:

Hussey, Jerry (MR #   ) Printed by   [   ] at 3/18/11... Page 2 of

from April 19, 2005, document (page 2)

"The pathologic features do not support a metastatic germ cell (testicular) tumor. . . . TTF-1 is a fairly specific lung cancer marker and B-HCG is well described in NSCCL (non-small cell carcinoma of the lung). We would not expect this degree of B-HCG in a seminoma (testicular germ cell tumor). . . . The pathology interpretation certainly suggests a recurrence of his lung carcinoma rather than his testicular carcinoma."

With all the documents I had reviewed, I appreciated that this report was relatively easy to understand, as written by Dr. PM, and finally, an *aha* moment, as it all started to come together. I smiled as I noticed he had CC'd both Dr. Lance and Dr. GP 2. What a relief to read the report that gave not only a definitive diagnosis, but also documented the science that substantiated it.

But even more than that, I smiled as I envisioned Dr. Lance reading it and cringing at the professional slap down. It felt like justice.

Jerry and I had been impressed with Dr. PM's professionalism when we'd met him, and thankfully, it seemed the newest oncologist had no tolerance for what appears to have been the incompetence of Dr. Lance.

Dr. PM had received and reviewed all Jerry's records before we met with him again. His notes reflected a definitive diagnosis based on Jerry's history and interpretation from the stains from the biopsy, rather than the feeble stance Dr. Lance had taken.

> There was positive staining for pancytokeratin, cytokeratin-7, beta HCG, and TTF-1. The presence of the TTF-1 is virtually diagnostic of lung or thyroid carcinoma. Given his prior history, this is certainly most compatible with recurrent lung carcinoma.

from April 19, 2005, document (page 3)

"The presence of the TTF-1 is virtually diagnostic of lung or thyroid carcinoma."

I lowered the paper to the table. There was no longer any other way to look at Dr. Lance's actions. Dr. PM's wording underscored the fact that *TTF-1 = lung or thyroid cancer* was apparently basic, elementary knowledge among oncologists. So, either Dr. Lance was largely incompetent as a cancer specialist, or he'd been willing to allow Jerry to be sent to Lance Armstrong's medical team, just so he might establish a relationship with the big boys.

Had he been willing to risk my Jerry's life in the hopes of a future promotion? Or, had he been incompetent in the extreme?

I pondered. Since Lance Armstrong's cancer team would have quickly found lung cancer in Jerry, just as Dr. PM had, that strongly indicated Dr. Lance had been stunningly incompetent.

Needing to know, I searched online for his name along with "doctor reviews." Twelve years had passed since Jerry and I had gone to see him, but recent reviews could still give me an idea of the oncologist's capabilities.

And at www.Vitals.com, I found these patient and family comments (slightly altered to avoid defamation issues, but otherwise intact).

- "[Dr. Lance] said my brother would be out of the hospital in a few days. Seven days later my brother died in tremendous pain."
- "I hope [Dr. Lance] learned something after the death of my daughter."
- "Disconnected from patient and their concerns. He doesn't heed warnings."
- "[Dr. Lance] neglected giving my wife the blood tests that he was required to. She died before she completed her treatment."
- "Very uncaring about my mother's fears."
- "If you have a cancerous tumor, don't stop here. Instead go to a university medical center. You may live longer."

I could only shake my head. These were, or had been, real people. Thank God that we now have the Internet and can check reviews before seeing a new doctor. And then we can leave reviews after a visit or experience. Had I been able at the time, I would have left reviews online myself, warning patients to steer clear of Dr. Lance.

As I moved on to the May 16, 2005, notes, and read the bottom third of page 4, unfortunately I had to doubt even Dr. PM's (or his transcribing staff's) competence.

Progress Notes signed by		at 05/16/05 1639	
Author:	Service:	(none)	Author Type: Advanced Practice Nurse
Filed: 05/16/05 1639	Note Time:	05/16/05 0927	

Cancer Center APN Follow up visit

Chief Compliant: Difficulty swallowing solids since Saturday. Week 3 of Carbo/Taxol with RT.

HPI: Mr. Hussey is seen today for follow up and chemotherapy. He has a history of lung and prostate cancer. He was diagnosed with lung cancer in Sept 2000. He underwent Carbo/VP=16. He

from May 16, 2005, document (page 4)

"Difficulty swallowing solids since Saturday." *Wrong!* The report completely minimized Jerry's symptoms. Jerry could not eat, drink, or swallow his own spit.

"He has a history of lung and prostate cancer."

How easily they get paperwork wrong. He never had prostate cancer. From this point on, Dr. PM's medical paperwork reads that Jerry had a history of lung and *prostate* cancer. Once they made that mistake on the documentation, it was copied and pasted onto all the paperwork in Dr. PM's office.

I found other important mistakes as well, including how many rounds of chemo Jerry had completed at a certain point.

But that is enough of medical records pertaining to cancer three. I realize that what I'm sharing may be a lot to process at first, but I believe people need to understand how botched conventional medical treatment can be, from hurried or incompetent doctors to mistakes in medical records.

If the painful discoveries I made while going through Jerry's documents in 2017 inspire you to read your own records and be your own advocate, then this year of hell will have been worth every moment.

☐

AHCC

On to a big positive. I thought it might be intriguing to research AHCC today, and what I found is compelling. Perhaps Dr. PM shouldn't have been so flippant about my recommendation, and Jerry's use of, AHCC mushroom supplement. The data is in, and it's well documented.

What follows are direct quotes from articles on the AHCC Research Association website.[15]

Research Summary

AHCC is the world's most researched specialty immune supplement, supported by over 20 human studies and by more than 100 pre-clinical *in vivo* and *in vitro* studies. It is utilized by over 1000 health care facilities worldwide to reduce the incidence of infections in both healthy and immune-compromised patients, improve cancer patient outcomes, decrease chemo side effects, help control HPV infections, manage viral loads in Hepatitis-C patients, and help those with liver disease.

AHCC has been used with great success in cancer patients. Data from the treatment of over 100,000 individuals with various types of cancer have shown AHCC treatment to be of benefit in 60 percent of cases (Kenner p. 15). AHCC is particularly effective for liver, lung, stomach, colon, breast, thyroid, ovarian, testicular, tongue, kidney, and pancreatic cancers (Kenner p. 15).

One landmark AHCC trial enrolled 269 patients with liver cancer. Following surgery, about half of the patients took AHCC and about half did not. The results were dramatic: At the end of the ten-year study, only 34.5 percent of the AHCC patients experienced a recurrence in their cancer, compared with 66.1 percent of the control group. Similarly, while 46.8 percent of the patients in the control group had died at the end of ten years, less than half that amount—20.4 percent—of those in the AHCC group had. Another study found that AHCC not only prolonged survival of advanced liver cancer patients, it also improved various parameters of quality of life, including mental stability,

---

[15] https://www.ahccresearch.org/

general physical health status, and the ability to have normal activities.

Chemotherapy is fraught with side effects, which range from psychologically distressing to life-threatening. In addition to being able to fight cancer directly, AHCC also alleviates many of the side effects of chemotherapy, including:

- **Hair Loss:** Doctors noticed that chemotherapy patients taking AHCC did not lose their hair. Subsequently, a study on mice found those treated with AHCC were protected from chemically induced hair loss.
- **Nausea:** Clinical studies in Korea and Japan have indicated that AHCC remarkably improves symptoms of nausea and vomiting in cancer patients (Kenner, p. 18). (As I recall, Jerry had little nausea while taking AHCC. We'd attributed it to the type of chemotherapy or an improvement in anti-nausea medicine.)
- **Bone Marrow Suppression:** Chemotherapy can inhibit bone marrow function, which is life-threatening because the body's key immune soldiers—the white blood cells—originate in bone marrow. AHCC has been shown to raise the white blood cell count of cancer patients by about 30 percent (Kenner, p. 17).
- **Liver Damage:** One of the major drawbacks of chemotherapy is that it kills healthy cells in addition to cancer cells. (Note that this places a tremendous burden on the liver.) An *in vivo* study found that while rats given chemotherapy experienced large increases in liver enzymes (indicative of liver damage), those given chemotherapy plus AHCC had normal levels (Kenner, p. 17).

I chuckle as I cynically wonder, is Dr. PM (Psychedelic Mushroom) one of the "over 1000 health care facilities worldwide" using this mushroom nutrient today? But in all seriousness, I do believe AHCC significantly contributed to

Jerry's recovery. After all, he enjoyed five years cancer-free in contrast to the four- to six-month terminal prognosis Dr. PM had given him.

However, cancer eventually showed up again.

Chapter 8
Hiatus

2006 to 2010

We finally made it through cancer number three and returned to a fairly normal life. Jerry continued to work in his woodshop creating beautiful furniture and gifts but didn't have the time to market his creations. He preferred to make custom pieces, and it was becoming an expensive hobby. We had all the furniture our home could accommodate, so his time spent in the shop diminished.

His truck driving career happily came to a screeching halt when a good friend and former supervisor called and asked Jerry to come to work for him. It was such a blessing. Jerry would be back in outside sales and traveling again, which he loved. Life was good!

Of course, Jerry and his friends enjoyed reminiscing whenever they got together. Back in the day . . . Invariably they would talk about the cars they'd had, and wished they still had—their first or favorite. Jerry had owned more than a dozen cars before he and I had met, but his favorites were a mountain green 1967 Camaro, and an orange 1970 Dodge Dart Swinger with a 340-cubic-inch engine and positraction.

With a desire to own a collector car, Jerry started researching what was available. At first I thought he was joking. He had a full woodworking shop, so where would he put a car? I chuckled and said to him, "The only difference between men and boys is the size and price of their toys."

But he was serious. I questioned whether we could afford it. He decided that he really didn't want to pay the going price for a decent Camaro or Swinger, and he wasn't looking for a show car. He wanted something he could tinker with and make his own, not an old beater either, just something to drive and have fun.

That led to a more serious conversation—truly, could we even afford it?

In a moment of complete candor, he said, "I have the money in my retirement account. I don't think I'll live long enough to enjoy retirement, so why can't I spend it on something I can enjoy now?"

Jerry had worked hard his whole life and had provided a good life for us. He'd made sacrifices by traveling all over the country, missing birthdays; the kids' soccer, baseball, and basketball games; and school activities, to support the family. I had to agree with him. He deserved it.

He found a 1965 Ford Mustang in good condition, though it needed some restoration. I understood he'd be compromising from the kind of car he really wanted (less than one-third the cost of a Camaro or Swinger). The Mustang was part of American car history and a connection to our youth. The nostalgia made us both smile, and we could afford it.

We hopped into my car to go see the Mustang.

Of course, when we both saw it, we were transported back in time. We took it for a test-drive and couldn't stop grinning. Naturally, we bought it. I drove my car home, and Jerry drove the Mustang.

Soon after, deliveries arrived in the form of Mustang magazines, boxes of chrome engine parts, an 8-track player, and other retro items. Occasionally we'd go to Mustang-parts businesses in the area looking for new wheels or other parts, and Jerry would occasionally visit junkyards while he was out traveling.

I thought back to our second year of marriage. Jerry had bought a 1959 MGA, and the two of us had restored it. Although we'd had a lot of fun working together on the MGA, I didn't join Jerry working on the Mustang. I had my own interests and commitments, but I loved our rides and seeing all the custom additions Jerry made, especially the 8-track player, dice door locks, and fuzzy dice hanging from the mirror. He, on the other hand, was more excited about the chrome additions to the engine, new mag wheels, and pinstriping he'd added.

We kept things positive, and we kept looking forward.

☐

Because Jerry traveled so much, I had been able to stave off getting a dog. We'd had them most of our marriage, and I loved them, but our kids were out on their own and so dog care chiefly fell on my shoulders. Inevitably, I was always the one to take the dogs in to be put to sleep. It had been a couple of years since our last dog, Tank, had to go for his last merciful shot.

One evening over dinner, Jerry broached the subject cautiously, about how much he missed having a dog, knowing full well what my response would be: they're so much work, the training, his travels, my schedule, the final trip to the vet. It was a tough conversation.

Then he set his fork on his plate, looked at me, and put it all on the line. "Diane, I just want a dog for companionship, to pet and to keep me company. I don't want a puppy. I want a dog that I can die with."

I wasn't prepared for that, and it tore me up. I said, "That's not fair!"

It *wasn't* fair! He didn't have cancer at the time (but it always seemed to be looming in the back of his mind), so that hit me out of the blue.

It wasn't fair, because I'd have to take care of the dog while he was out of town, feeding him and letting him out throughout the day amid my work schedule. And invariably Jerry was out of town when the grass needed cutting, so I'd have to pick up after the dog as well.

It wasn't fair, because—being completely practical—if Jerry died before the dog did, I'd have to continue to take care of the dog, for how long? And, eventually, when the dog got so old and sick that it needed to go to the vet for the final shot, I'd be a wreck again, like I had been with all our previous dogs.

Jerry said, "I'd really like another German Shorthaired Pointer."

We'd had one, and our daughter, Tara, had one as well. They both had a lot of character.

Jerry resumed eating. "I've been doing a little research and found a local German Shorthair rescue organization."

The conversation continued. Ultimately, I conceded.

Before he'd been rescued, our new dog, Connor, had been running the streets during winter. Afraid of everyone, he had avoided being caught for months. By the time rescuers captured him, he was emaciated, had heartworm, and had lost the hair on his ears from frostbite.

It took months after Connor was rescued before he could be adopted. First his medical requirements had to be fulfilled at the veterinarian's office, and then he'd gone on to a loving foster home for months of rehab.

It was heartbreaking to see how scared Connor was of everyone and nearly everything. He cowered and hid under Jerry's desk and would hide under the kitchen table waiting for the back door to open, so he could run outside. When he came in, Connor would hide under the kitchen table waiting for the coast to clear, so he could run upstairs and hide under the desk.

Although I was guilted into getting a dog, I must admit that Connor was good for Jerry, and Jerry was good for Connor.

At night, he'd sleep on the floor by Jerry. When Jerry was traveling, Connor would sleep in that same place, awaiting his return. Connor tolerated me when Jerry was out of town, and I confess, I really didn't want the heartbreak of getting close to Connor.

Over the years, Connor did grow to have a personality under Jerry's patient encouragement, and the special bond of unconditional love grew between them that animal lovers understand.

☐

As I've mentioned, Jerry and I didn't argue. That wasn't our nature, either of us. As I reflect on this time in our lives, I want to be candid: We had a good marriage, loved each other with a deep love, and were settled into a comfortable routine. However, like many others, we fell into a rut over the years, taking each other for granted.

To put the car and dog conversations into perspective, I'd like to draw upon wisdom learned from the book *The 5 Love Languages* by Gary Chapman.

My love language was "acts of service," which basically meant I showed love by what I did. For Jerry, my acts of service at this time included all the typical household chores, but also shoveling snow, cutting the grass, and doing whatever I could to make his life easier and better. So, of course, I would take care of Connor for Jerry. Because I loved him, I would do whatever I could to make him happy.

The love language we speak or do is the same as what we would like to receive, so I wanted Jerry to do things for me without being asked.

Jerry's love language was "words of affirmation." He frequently told me how much he loved me and how wonderful I was—not as a ploy to get something, he was just very good at verbally expressing his feelings and love.

Because I had a different love language, Jerry's words didn't touch me as deeply or have the impact he'd expected. He wanted to hear how wonderful he was, and how much I appreciated all that he did. Until I read *The 5 Love Languages*, which was sometime after we got the Mustang and Connor, I never realized how important words were—I was busy *showing* Jerry how much I loved him while he was *telling* me how much he loved me.

If we'd read that book by this time, I'm guessing we would have appreciated each other more, not feeling like we'd been going through the motions and passing like proverbial ships in the night. We got the car. We got Connor. We got along. But we weren't fully understanding each other.

Some may wonder why I share these things that have little to do with cancer. A friend told me about Chapman's book, and I truly appreciated what I learned about Jerry and myself. It helped me put some of my struggles into perspective as I began to understand why we did what we did.

Cancer is more than the physical battle. If we can identify some of our relationship issues (impacting our mental and emotional health), it may help us in our overall journey.

□

During this time I moved on from selling cars into selling life insurance and annuities. I still couldn't figure out what to be when I grew up but knew I didn't want a "job." I had more of an entrepreneurial spirit and had enjoyed helping seniors as a caregiver. Incorporating my accounting/financial background with a desire to assist them in protecting their family's finances and retirement seemed a good choice.

I also developed a deeper hunger for knowing God and cultivating a strong relationship with Him. I began to spend considerable time pursuing God through prayer, reading the Bible, studying, and becoming involved in a small ministry.

In addition to the ministry, our group shared an interest in natural health. Collectively we started to make changes to improve our overall well-being.

In 2009, one of my friends discovered the benefits of Enagic's Kangen Water®, the premier ionic water system that changes the properties of water to make it more alkaline.

Cancer can't live in an oxygen-rich/alkaline-rich environment, so it made sense to me to purchase the water system for our health, especially with Jerry's cancer history. He couldn't be convinced of the health benefits of drinking Kangen Water, and wouldn't take the time to research it, so he continued to consume his favorite beverages: coffee, iced tea, and beer, which are all acidic.

Jerry had his Mustang to work on and a traditional job, while I was focusing on God, ministry, and essentially starting my own business. We still loved each other, with strong bonds that continued to hold us together, but much of the time it seemed like we were each involved in our own individual activities. The more we pursued our own interests, the less time we spent doing things together.

Love hadn't dimmed. Simply, busyness had gradually taken over.

It hurts me to think about it, but God was about to change that, as Jerry would soon be diagnosed with his fourth cancer and then his fifth. We'd been such a great team early on in our marriage, and we were still great together working on major home improvement projects. But as great as we'd been in the past, we were about to become an even better and stronger team with the battle before us.

Chapter 9
Cancer Four

2010

Jerry and I busily cruised along through life. When the retaining wall next to the driveway shifted, we removed and replaced it. We were always at our best when we worked on projects together.

Jerry was still out selling, traveling to see clients and distributors weekdays, and home working on the Mustang weekends with Connor curled up nearby.

In October 2010, I started taking natural health classes at New Eden School of Natural Health & Herbal Studies,[16] along with a couple of friends who shared the desire to live a healthier lifestyle. It would take months of intense study to earn my Natural Health Counselor certification.

☐

2011

Thankfully, five years had gone by since Jerry finished treatment for his third cancer. Had the AHCC, the daily mushroom supplement, been a contributing factor? I believe so, and Jerry took it every day, likewise convinced that it made a difference.

He had dutifully kept his doctor appointments with Dr. PM for blood work and CT scans. It seemed Jerry always had an underlying concern that if he didn't feel well the cancer was returning. As I understand it, that reaction is, sadly, common among those who've had the disease. But for the most part he felt healthy and happy.

Everything seemed to be going well until January 2011 when Jerry visited Dr. PM for his semiannual checkup. As always, he weighed in, had blood drawn, and was escorted to the exam room. But this time, the doctor walked in with a mild look of concern. Jerry's platelet count, which should be about 150,000 in the average male, was at 90,000.

Platelet counts can be affected by a variety of factors, the doctor said. Although the 40 percent loss in platelets was significant, it must not have been

---

[16] https://www.newedenschoolofnaturalhealth.org/

too disconcerting to the doctor. He scheduled Jerry to come back in two weeks to recheck the blood work.

Again, Jerry's platelets dropped, plus questions arose about other components of his blood.

Dr. PM asked Jerry to return one month later for yet another blood draw. He also told Jerry to make a few dietary changes and ordered a few other tests to try to home in on the reason his platelets continued to drop.

Since the oncologist didn't seem overly concerned, we weren't either.

☐

While Jerry underwent the monthly blood tests, I finished up my natural health classes and certification. I had already completed the classes Anatomy and Physiology, Natural Health and Nutrition, Natural Health Approaches, Herbology, and Herbal First Aid.

My friend and classmate, Melissa, enjoyed the same hunger for learning that I did. We devoured information and tore through the classes, challenging each other on understanding and recollection. We both finished our coursework for the CNHC (Certified Natural Health Counselor) in record time, and both passed with straight A's.

Excited, I wanted to share all that I was learning about natural health with Jerry, but he remained less than receptive to hearing about it. We didn't know what exact issues had arisen with his blood work, but the doctor had an eye on it. Although I hadn't received specific schooling on blood work, it seemed important to me that we make some changes to improve Jerry's immune system, because a strong immune system is critical to maintaining good health.

I suggested he drink the ionized Kangen Water since cancer cannot live in an alkaline environment. I also recommended he change up his diet to include more nature-based foods and fewer processed foods so that he'd have a higher intake of nutrients that energized, strengthened, and healed.

Jerry remained contrary on both, despite the documented science. It's sad to say, but people like Jerry who need natural health methods in order to build their immune systems are often the most resistant. Instead, they rely on conventional doctors and medications with their many side effects.

To that point, the most compelling research I'd found regarding basic natural approaches for people with cancer, or who are at risk for cancer, is to eat healthy (preferably organic) foods, increase the body's alkalinity, reduce stress, get plenty of exercise and rest, and get rid of the toxins poisoning their bodies, part of which are their food and beverage choices.

I must confess that occasionally I became angry with Jerry because he didn't take care of himself. He ate and drank all the wrong things and wasn't willing to make changes. We didn't quite stand at opposite ends of the spectrum on health, but close. Occasionally he would mock the changes I made trying to be healthier, which created a bit of a chasm between us.

⬜

At Jerry's next appointment at the end of February, his blood work seriously concerned Dr. PM. His platelets had dropped significantly, and the doctor immediately ordered a bone marrow biopsy.

A couple of weeks elapsed while Jerry scheduled and underwent the bone marrow biopsy, and a few days more while the results were forwarded to Dr. PM. Our next appointment was scheduled for early March.

To say that we felt anxious during the hour-plus drive to Dr. PM's office for the biopsy results would be an understatement. Somehow, I think we both sensed a dark cloud hovering over us.

There was no focusing on the unusual objects in the doctor's office. We were consumed with learning the truth.

From the moment he entered the room, Dr. PM's demeanor alone told us we were in for a sobering conversation. He picked up the results of the biopsy and tried to ease into the conversation. But all of that became a blur when I heard "blood cancer."

I asked him to slow down and repeat what he had just said. I wanted to take notes about the diagnosis.

He repeated, "Jerry has myelodysplastic syndrome, MDS, a blood cancer."

Wait, I thought. *Jerry doesn't have any major symptoms, only the changes in blood work. Though,* I vaguely recalled, *a lack of symptoms isn't uncommon for many who are diagnosed with cancer.*

Unlike our previous conversations with oncologists, where they usually seemed to have good news to go with the bad, this time there was no good news. Only bad.

The doctor leaned back in his chair, as if to impart a calmness over the situation.

Jerry's thumb stroked the arm of his chair, unconsciously using the touch for self-comfort. "What do you recommend for treatment?"

My pen hovered over my notepaper.

"The normal treatment consists of ten straight days of injections, including weekends, and then eighteen days off. Then another ten days on, eighteen days off. This will continue for at least six months."

My thoughts raced, struggling to comprehend what the doctor was saying, while also trying to imagine how we were going to incorporate that schedule into our lives.

Dr. PM continued, "The second option is a new, experimental program that adds a pill. The pill is expected to enhance the results of the standard treatment. The shot regiment remains the same."

Dr. PM made it seem so simple: Here are your options. Injections without pill, injections with pill. Done.

My pen wrote a few notes. Then I asked, "What are your thoughts about adding natural health supplements to strengthen Jerry's immune system, and whether that might help Jerry's platelet issue?"

Jerry slanted me a look like, *What are you trying to do? He's the doctor.*

The doctor pooh-poohed my question and then turned toward Jerry, dismissing me like I had no idea what I was talking about.

As with most pharmaceutical-based doctors (MDs), Dr. PM was still unreceptive to anything nature-based that I'd learned about and now advocated. On occasion he'd continued to mock AHCC as "psychedelic mushrooms."

Refocus, Diane.

Completely ignoring the fact that I'd been dismissed, I spoke up again. "What can Jerry expect from the treatment? What drugs would he be receiving, and what are their side effects?"

Curiously, Dr. PM started tap-dancing. "Well, this isn't really chemo." He paused as if searching for the right words. "Instead of infusions that take hours to administer, Jerry will just receive a shot each time. And if there are side effects, they won't be the life-altering chemotherapy reactions he's experienced previously. They will be very mild. And he'll receive the injections here at the hospital, and at the affiliated hospital down the road on weekends."

Dr. PM steered our focus to the experimental program, and the expected enhancement of the combined medications. "The cycle will continue for six months, minimum," Dr. PM reiterated, "and up to twenty-four months."

Jerry sighed and looked at me. "That's a daunting schedule. Ten days in a row. We live at least an hour and fifteen minutes from the hospital, up to two hours during rush hour. And that's one way."

The doctor said, "Jerry, you could start your day with the shot and go on to work afterward."

Jerry was still looking at me, gauging my thoughts. "It would make for very long workdays, Diane. And on weekends I'd be looking at a minimum three-hour drive round-trip, just to get a shot. That would mean a lot of driving time, time spent away from work and home." Jerry looked over at the doctor. "Can this be done through our local hospital?"

I'd just been thinking the same.

Dr. PM shook his head. "No. This treatment is experimental. It'll have to be done here."

My mind circled back around to the doctor's statement, *"This isn't really chemo."* I asked, "Is it, or is it not, chemotherapy?"

"Well, technically the medication is chemo—"

We both voiced concern at the same time. "Jerry already had too much chemo. You told us that when you stopped Jerry's chemo treatment with his third cancer."

The doctor held up a hand to halt our objection. "The amount that Jerry would be receiving is minimal, and he should have few, if any, side effects."

Again I thought how Jerry hadn't been able to receive all the chemo that Dr. PM himself had prescribed for his third cancer. And now he wanted to give him more? It didn't make sense, and I couldn't help but think natural, holistic health made far more sense. Jerry and I would have to discuss that option, but later, not in front of the doctor.

I made myself ask, "What can we expect in terms of life expectancy?"

"Maybe two and a half years. But this experimental program is considered the best course of treatment for MDS at this time."

Maybe.

Experimental.

Up to three hours of driving per day.

I asked Jerry, "What kind of quality of life would we have?"

His blue eyes locked on mine, as if he'd been thinking the same.

It was all I could do to muster the courage to ask my final question. "And if we did nothing?"

"Maybe six months."

Jerry took my hand and held it in both of his. His warm grip gave strength as much as sought it. "Diane, I don't know if it's worth it."

"But wait!" Dr. PM suddenly leaned forward, drawing both our gazes. "It's your opportunity to help others! They can use the research to help future cancer patients!"

Really? I thought. *You're applying guilt to try to turn my Jerry into a lab rat?* Jerry and I had known people who'd gotten caught in that trap, and their last few years or months had been horrible.

Dr. PM's hands gestured earnestly as he went on about advancements in research and new treatments and therapies. But my mind had shifted and wasn't absorbing what he was saying. *When we get home, I'll need to research MDS, blood cancer, and natural health therapies for it online.*

Retrieving my purse, I filed away my notebook and pen. Dr. PM's experimental plan, in his words, had been, *"The best course of treatment."* My unstated thoughts: *I don't think so.*

Jerry said, "We'll consider what you've told us and get back to you."

Dr. PM gave Jerry the packet of information about the experimental treatment program, the last page of which, he pointed out, was the consent form.

☐

The fourth cancer. We walked out of the office in silence, each processing in our own way all that had been said.

Jerry called his boss to let him know he wouldn't be in to work that afternoon. He briefly told him about the blood cancer diagnosis, and that we needed time to consider our options.

We stopped for lunch at one of our favorite restaurants. There was no need for a menu. We knew what we wanted. It was what we always ordered. Jerry had barbequed ribs, and I ordered Oriental chicken salad.

As we sat there, the silence was deafening. We were numb, and in shock, as we tried to process what we'd heard, one of us asking partial questions, the other completing the thoughts.

The treatment, being experimental, seemed highly suspect, at best.

And with what quality of life? Just the schedule alone was disconcerting. It would consume our lives.

And the chemotherapy? Sure, it was only an injection, and far less than what Jerry had received through the IVs he'd had previously, but he'd already undergone sixty doses of chemo. He hadn't even been able to finish his last chemo treatment because his body had no longer been able to tolerate it.

We picked at our lunches, realizing we really weren't very hungry, and that nothing would taste good anyway.

I don't believe either of us really gave much thought to the lifespan Dr. PM had mentioned. To us, it wasn't acceptable. At all.

□

We left the restaurant, started driving, each retreating again into our own thoughts. Finally, Jerry broke the silence. "Ten days of shots followed by eighteen days off. The time and distance. For an unknown quality of life. For an unknown period of time. With unknown side effects."

I said, "Dr. PM tap-danced around the chemotherapy and side-effects question."

"I think he did too. And did he seem eager to you to get me into the experimental treatment program?"

"Yes. Very."

Jerry tilted his head, acknowledging our mutual agreement. "That option isn't worth it. It's time to seek a second opinion."

We *were* going to move forward, and an unproven, experimental version of chemo wasn't an option we were willing to settle for. We would seek something else.

Still, a fourth cancer . . .

I started to choke up. "Jerry, we need to call the kids. Tonight." We didn't like the diagnosis, and weren't willing to accept the doctor's prognosis, but we did need to let our children know what was going on.

Jerry agreed.

They would be three really difficult calls.

"We should probably go visit my parents to break the news to them in person," I said softly.

"Makes sense. We'll visit them this weekend."

As before, we each drifted into our own little world, neither saying much. My mother and aunts are masters of worrying. It's as if they try to figure out every possible scenario, and it ties them up in emotional knots. Jerry and I were more likely to think things through, anticipating and logically problem solving, like in a chess game.

Jerry had mentioned getting a second opinion. Me? I would focus on finding alternatives to anything considered to be conventional medical treatment.

When we got home, Jerry again called his boss and good friend, confessing what we had discussed and letting him know we would be seeking a second opinion.

I, on the other hand, started researching online. There wasn't much to find about MDS. The little I located was that MDS may be referred to as a pre-leukemia or a bone marrow failure disorder, and the prognosis was bleak. It seemed to me the odds were stacked against Jerry. I shuddered.

Again, I typed, altering search terms. Well, it appeared the medical community was learning more about blood cancers, with a focus on distinguishing the differences and methods of treatment.

Hm. In natural health, the focus was on finding and dealing with not merely the issue, but also the source of the issue, which, in my dandelion analogy, was whatever caused the seeds/cells to grow. So, how might we give Jerry's body the ability to heal itself—to get rid of even the cancer cells—by improving his immune system and giving his body what it needed?

I didn't want Jerry treated. I wanted him healed.

As I continued to search online, I discovered Cancer Tutor (www.CancerTutor.com), a fantastic resource with all sorts of options. I found something called the Budwig Diet, information about detoxing, beneficial nutrients, cellular energy, alkalinity, and several protocols worthy of consideration and implementation. The options were promising.

Just one small wrinkle. Not only was I going to have to convince Jerry, but the kids as well.

That evening, we called Brandon, Devin, and Tara, having managed to pull it together before dialing. They all wanted to come up from Texas and assured us they'd arrange to get off work and be up within the week. We told them they didn't have to, but they all insisted. Naturally they were upset and needed reassurance. They needed to see and hear their dad in person.

At least now as a distributor for Enagic's Kangen Water ionizers and also scalar energy devices, I could choose my hours. I was available for family time, appointments, and anything Jerry might need.

Online, Cancer Tutor became one of my go-to resources. I tried sharing with Jerry all that I was learning. He might "listen" to humor me, but Jerry remained skeptical about anything I turned up while researching or had learned in my classes (other than his belief in AHCC). Jerry trusted doctors. After all, doctors had gone to *medical* school and had degrees and experience. In his eyes I was just a novice, so how could I possibly know anything that the doctors and medical system didn't?

It's amazing to me how God works. I believe the small incident that was about to take place created another crack to open Jerry's eyes to natural health options.

Jerry came into the kitchen one morning complaining of a headache.

A bit testy, I thought, *What do you want me to do about it?* Why didn't he just take an aspirin or other pain reliever like he normally would? It can be very tiresome to provide multiple alternatives to an issue and have them all be rejected, but I offered my scalar energy pendant (I'll explain the science shortly) to him and told him to rub it wherever it hurt.

He'd been a complete skeptic when I'd tried to explain the benefits to him previously, so he responded, "You do it," like a child.

I sighed and rubbed the pendant where he pointed on his forehead.

His headache lessened, and he went back upstairs.

About fifteen minutes later, he came back down and said, "Try that again."

We repeated the procedure.

About fifteen minutes later he came down again and said, "I'll try wearing one of those things."

I had tried since December to share what I'd learned about scalar energy and its health benefits with Jerry, but he hadn't been interested until now, when he'd unwittingly opened the door to the possibility.

Scalar energy can protect us from negative electrical energy sources (mobile phones, computers, Wi-Fi—pretty much everything electrical and electronic) and help relieve pain, among other things.

In my natural health classes, I'd learned that cancer cells are low-energy cells, and by increasing the cellular energy, cancer cells have been shown to revert to normal. There's a lot more to it, but that's what I'd been trying to impart to Jerry. I had learned over the years not to inundate him with details, but to offer just enough of the big picture to pique his curiosity. Hopefully, he'd start to research for himself at some point.

That morning, Jerry started wearing a scalar energy pendant regularly.

The next time Jerry had his blood checked, his platelets had dropped by only 2,000 per week instead of 4,500 per week as they had previously. We told Dr. PM about the pendant and scalar energy, but of course he expressed complete skepticism.

Based on the blood test results, Jerry asked for a second scalar energy device when we got home. I dug out a bracelet and prayed for improvement and healing.

At his next appointment, his platelets had dropped by just 1,000 per week. Afterward, his platelets remained stable for months.

When we again mentioned scalar energy to the doctor, he didn't say anything.

I asked, "Is it normal for platelets to level off like that?"

He said, "No."

I explained the research behind scalar energy, since that was the only thing Jerry had changed.

The doctor had no answer.

My impression? The oncologist wasn't open to anything other than the medical establishment (pharmacy-based) modalities.

It seemed, during this conversation, that Jerry likewise developed the opinion that very few doctors listen to alternative therapies, just as Jerry hadn't listened to me, until he'd experienced the benefits of natural approaches firsthand.

Dr. PM's response caused a significant fracture in Jerry's confidence in his oncologist's receptivity of anything outside of chemo, radiation, and surgery—literally poisoning, burning, and cutting.

Moreover, Dr. PM increasingly displayed an overbearing attitude that he had *THE* way, the *ONLY* way, that MDS must be treated.

From that day forward, every time something new came up, Jerry observed that the oncologist wasn't willing to listen, even to proven and documented science of alternative methods of healing.

□

The Science: Scalar Energy

So why am I excited about scalar energy? I learned about scalar energy in my natural health classes when our class attended a demonstration on scalar energy products, shortly before Jerry was diagnosed with MDS. Scalar products, often found in the form of necklace pendants or bracelets, are designed to protect us from the electromagnetic frequencies (EMFs) that we are constantly exposed to through electrical and electronic devices. I was fascinated by the science and presentation.

While I realize that some things are best explained during a demonstration, that isn't possible here, so hopefully this will give you a foundational understanding.

The Problem—EMFs

Our bodies are bombarded with electromagnetic frequencies (EMFs) from mobile phones, televisions, computers, Wi-Fi, automobiles, microwaves, our refrigerators, everything electrical and electronic. Never in all of history have our bodies been under such attack. (*Please* do yourself a favor and watch the six-minute video *Microwave Radiation Dangers in Your Home*,[17] featuring Dr. Magda Havas, PhD, for greater understanding about the threats of EMFs to our health. The term *microwave* in the video title does not refer to the unit that cooks food, but to the form of waves that pose danger to us all.)

How are EMFs detrimental to our health? EMFs cause our blood cells to clump together like stacked coins. When blood cells stick together, it clogs blood vessels, interferes with the delivery of oxygen and nutrients and the removal of wastes, and so it creates very unhealthy blood. In another video, Magda Havas states, "A doctor told me this (clumping of the blood cells) is what she sees with cancer patients."

While the videos featuring Magda Havas are effective for understanding the impact of EMFs on our bodies, the problem has been tremendously exacerbated by advances in technology with 5G technology and smart meters.

5G technology is being rolled out across the U.S. while global resistance is mounting over health concerns. Our bodies are not designed to handle the EMF assault.

Smart meters emit 160 times more cumulative whole-body exposure than a cell phone and have been linked to numerous health issues, including:

- cancer
- learning and memory problems
- difficulty sleeping

---

[17] https://www.youtube.com/watch?v=aAnrmJ3un1g

- fatigue
- tinnitus
- headaches
- anxiety and depression
- arthritis
- skin reaction
- hyperactivity in children
- neuropathy[18]

The Science

James Clark Maxwell, a Scottish mathematical genius whose work led to the development of quantum physics and is best known for his formulation of electromagnetic theory, first proposed the existence of scalar energy in the mid-1800s. Nearly fifty years later, Nicola Tesla, generally considered the father of scalar electromagnetics, was able to demonstrate scalar energy, and began to harness scalar energy without using wires. He referred to it as standing energy or universal waves, and his name for it was "radiant energy." His Tesla flat coil, which can produce scalar impulses, was patented January 9, 1894—patent #512340.[19] Even Albert Einstein and Otto Stern (physicist nominated eighty-two times for the Nobel Prize) acknowledged this form of energy in the 1920s.

Scalar energy can be created naturally, has always existed in the universe, is infinite, and by applying the conditions required, can also be created artificially.[20]

Unfortunately, when Tesla died, he took the secret of scalar generation with him, and almost another full century passed before science was once again able to positively demonstrate the existence of scalar energy and resume looking at its potential.

Scalar energy is unique. Since it is non-linear and non-Hertzian, it cannot be measured by contemporary frequency instruments. It has the capacity to carry information and does not decay with the passing of time or distance. It can pass through solid objects without losing intensity and can be embedded into products.

Our traditional understanding of energy is that it flows out in the form of waves. However, scalar energy does not radiate in the same way. Scalar

---

[18] https://thetruthaboutcancer.com/electric-smart-meters/
[19] www.quantumspanner.com/tesla—father-of-scalar-energy.html
[20] https://www.spooky2scalar.com/history-of-scalar-energy/

waves are described as three-dimensional waves that spin in a clockwise motion and can regenerate and repair itself indefinitely. Its shape is very similar to the structure of DNA as it folds in and around itself.[21] It is like a field of energy systems that is alive, a vibrant and dynamic energy field that radiates a network of harmoniously balanced energies.[22]

Volcanic rock, primarily from Japan and Iceland,[23] are the main sources for scalar energy products. They emit high levels of negative ions.

Why is that important?

Anything using electricity gives off positive ions, which can be transmitted to your body via EMFs. Each piece of household and office electrical equipment that radiates at 60 Hz interferes with our brain, nervous system, and individual cells in our body. Too many positive ions can cause damage at the cellular level and lead to health problems, including cancer.

The scalar energy devices worn for protection can also transfer scalar energy into food, drink, and supplements. Shields are available for mobile phones, computers, and similar electronic devices. Scalar energy can regenerate and repair itself indefinitely, so a device never wears out.

Now, taking all that and distilling it into an ultra-simplified explanation: Scalar energy products basically harness the earth's natural energy to provide a protective shield around the body that essentially removes and cancels the effects of man-made frequencies (60 Hz) on the human body.[24]

The Benefits

What health benefits are possible by exposing the human body to beneficial scalar energy frequencies?

- Scalar energy raises the vibratory frequency of anything placed within its field, including the blood of your body and water of your cells.
- Scalar energy improves cell wall permeability so the cells can eliminate waste and receive oxygen and nutrients more efficiently.
- Scalar energy is capable of imprinting itself on your DNA.
- Scalar waves have a pair of identical but opposing waves, which carry information and travel in a clockwise rotation.

---

[21] http://www.lasotaenergy.dk/wp-content/uploads/2014/11/Dokumentation-4.pdf
[22] http://www.lasotaenergy.dk/wp-content/uploads/2014/11/Dokumentation-4.pdf
[23] https://www.scalarenergypendants.com/
[24] http://www.lasotaenergy.dk/wp-content/uploads/2014/11/Dokumentation-4.pdf

- Our DNA rotates in a clockwise motion, allowing scalar energy a harmonious assimilation with our cells.[25]
- A scalar energy device placed around consumable foods and liquids will transfer energy field frequencies to that food or liquid.
- It increases our overall body energy levels as a result of increasing the cellular energy.
- It is proven in laboratory studies to improve immune function.
- It improves mental focus (as measured by EEG frequencies).
- It balances the two hemispheres of the brain (as measured by EEG tests).[26]

Dr. Jon Barron postulates: Cancer cells are, almost without exception, low-voltage cells operating at 15 to 20 millivolts, whereas a normal cell is in the 70 to 90 millivolt range. One of the theories is that as cellular voltage drops into the range where the very survival of the cell may be in jeopardy, the cell begins to multiply uncontrollably in an attempt to survive. If we are able to raise the voltage, the cell no longer needs to proliferate uncontrollably, and can become "normal" again.[27]

His hypothesis is controversial, but I found it a logical one, based on the science behind it.

For those interested in researching further, scalar energy studies have been done related to improving sleep, cardiovascular benefits, relieving asthma and other respiratory problems, viral infection protection, and help with depression.

I am a huge proponent of scalar energy and continue to wear my pendant every day. It's a joy to demonstrate the protective effects, and a relief to know I'm protecting myself and my health.

☐

Shortly after Jerry was diagnosed with cancer the fourth time, I received my credentials as a Certified Natural Health Counselor. The education was invaluable in understanding how the body works—disease and illness, the

---

[25] This and the preceding bulleted points are information found at http://freqe1.com/the-scalar-factor/scalar-waves/
[26] This and the preceding bulleted points are information found at https://jonbarron.org/article/energy-life.
[27] https://jonbarron.org/article/energy-life

immune system (getting healthy and staying healthy), and supplementation, to name a few. We were at a crossroads, and Jerry's health was on the line. He would be the one to make the ultimate decision regarding the course of treatment, but I was going to sneak in all the information I could.

Chapter 10
Summer 2017—The Quest for Truth:
Cancer Four

Grabbing the file for cancer four, I went into the living room and sat on the sofa. I looked around at Jerry's hand-crafted bookshelf, the matching corner cabinet, foyer bench, table, mirror, and the decorative storage boxes he had hand-pieced together. All of that was in the living room alone. I loved the patience and talent of the man.

My father had always been very handy, and while growing up I'd often helped him with projects. Jerry had been raised on a farm where he'd learned how to build and fix just about everything. Throughout our marriage Jerry and I had been able to do all types of projects together: roofing, plumbing, electrical, painting, wallpapering, laying a one-hundred-foot-long concrete sidewalk, jacking up a house to replace a rotten sill plate, replacing patio doors, installing windows, and building or repairing retaining walls, to name some of our projects completed.

Truly a great team! But the handmade furniture was all Jerry's baby, just as the interest in natural health was mine.

Sifting. Contrast. Light/dark. Truth/lies. Good/evil. The reminder drew my attention back to the file. My journey through the medical records for cancers one through three had been almost more than I could bear. I prayed that the medical records for cancer four wouldn't put me on the roller coaster of emotions again. I took a deep breath before opening and paging through the documents related to cancer four.

On Jerry's January 27, 2011, paperwork Dr. PM had noted, "Jerry has been disease free and off all treatment for over five years." I guess Dr. PM was able to say that since Jerry had survived the lung cancer in the lymph node, but cancer had reared its ugly head again, this time in the blood, so could the doctor really claim victory?

During my research I've learned that the American Cancer Society and the rest of the medical establishment no longer talk about a "cure." Instead, they refer to a five-year relative survival rate. Who decided, and how was it decided, that five years would be the target time frame? Why not seven years? Or ten years? Is it because the medical community knew the statistics and had to lower the bar to five years to give us a false sense of victory? I like how naturopathic doctor Dr. Peter Glidden points out in his video *Chemotherapy Is a Waste of Money*[28] that their goal is no longer a cure, but about reaching the magic "five years" . . . and one day.

People I know want a cure. If they knew the doctor was looking to get them five years and one day, because that's become the revised goal, how many might reconsider their options? And how many might reconsider contributing to organizations that have lowered the bar from hope for a cure . . . to hope for five years and one day?

"Jerry has been disease free and off all treatment for over five years."

I stared at Dr. PM's comment. "Well, take a bow for surpassing the magic five-year mark," I muttered.

With a shake of my head, I moved on to the lab results from Jerry's February 28, 2011, testing date.

Hussey, Jerry (MR #   )

FISH Results: ABNORMAL MYELODYSPLASTIC SYNDROME PANEL, POSITIVE FOR DELETION 5q AND DELETION 7q

Fluorescence in situ hybridization (FISH) analysis was performed with Vysis probes specific for chromosome 5 (D5S721, D5S23, EGR1), chromosome 7 (D7Z1, D7S486), the pericentromeric region of chromosome 8 (D8Z2), and the long arm of chromosome 20 (D20S108).

Two hundred nuclei were examined for each chromosome. The signal patterns obtained for chromosome 5 demonstrated one hundred thirty-five cells with a loss of EGR1 gene, indicating a deletion in the long arm. The probe for chromosome 7 showed forty-eight cells with a loss of D7S486 gene, indicating a deletion in the long arm. The remaining probes did not differ substantially from the normal control. Both del(5q) and del(7q) are associated with myeloid disorders.

The FISH tests for chromosomes 5, 7, and 20 were developed and their performance characteristics validated by   Systems. They have not been cleared or approved by the U.S. Food and Drug Administration. The probe for chromosome 8 has been FDA cleared.

from February 28, 2011, document (page 4)

I read through the highly complex assessment of this biopsy. Truly amazing, the medical community's ability to test for such specific indicators in the blood and bone marrow! The report stated, "Two hundred nuclei were examined for each chromosome. . . . The probe for chromosome 7 showed forty-eight cells with a loss of D7S486 gene."

With all of this technology, why is there no cure for cancer? Seriously! The ability of scientists to isolate and analyze this type of information is staggering.

For all the time, energy, and money thrown at cancer, where are the results?

---

[28] https://www.youtube.com/watch?v=XdLyMhNdcSc

The research seems impressive, but is it? Or is it just a shell game? Is the medical community making progress or just creating an illusion of busily studying and making claims to raise more money?

I often talk with people about cancer and the medical community. The tide seems to be turning as the public gains awareness. Many agree that the medical industry doesn't want a cure for cancer because there's just too much money at stake.

But I digress.

Needing to clearly understand MDS, since I've never fully understood it, I grabbed my laptop and searched online.

MDS is complicated by the fact that there are primary MDS and secondary or therapy-related MDS. That means many cancer patients who have received chemo treatment or radiation are at risk of developing this cancer in the future. The MDS Foundation website has excellent videos that keep primary and secondary MDS simple and understandable. One of the best videos I found for this was *Animation—Understanding Myelodysplastic Syndromes*.[29]

I felt grateful for the video since it finally helped me understand the severity of Jerry's MDS from the moment he was diagnosed. Although this is after the fact, it helps put everything in perspective.

I find myself caught in a quandary between wanting to cite scientific information or keeping it simple. My goal from the beginning has been to make cancer understandable to empower you, the reader. Hopefully by now I've gained your trust that what I present is well researched and truthful, so I am opting for simple explanations and recommending that anyone who wants more information about MDS search online. The MDS Foundation is a great resource, as are the American Cancer Society and the American Society of Hematology.

So, what exactly is MDS?

"Myelodysplastic Syndromes (MDS) are a group of diverse bone marrow disorders in which the bone marrow does not produce enough healthy blood cells."[30] MDS can occur when the blood-forming cells in the bone marrow become abnormal, which affects our body's ability to produce the components needed for healthy blood and leads to low numbers of red blood cells, white blood cells, and/or platelets.

Abnormal blood cells, characterized by uncontrolled growth, multiply rapidly crowding out our body's ability to create strong, vigorous and normal

[29] http://www.youandmds.com/en-mds/view/m101-a01-understanding-myelodysplastic-syndromes-animation
[30] https://www.mds-foundation.org/what-is-mds

blood cells that would normally transport oxygen, fight off serious infections, or prevent serious bleeding.

(Below, I use *italics* to highlight aspects directly attributed to Jerry's cancer.)

> What causes MDS? With a few exceptions, the exact causes of MDS are unknown. . . . *Radiation and chemotherapy for cancer are among the known triggers for the development of MDS.* Patients who take chemotherapy drugs or who receive radiation therapy for potentially curable cancers, such as breast or *testicular cancers*, Hodgkin's disease and non-Hodgkin's lymphoma, *are at risk of developing MDS for up to ten years following treatment. MDS that develops after use of cancer chemotherapy or radiation is called "secondary MDS"* and is usually associated with multiple chromosome abnormalities in cells in the bone marrow.[31]

Equipped with the knowledge that chemotherapy can cause MDS, it would be helpful to know which types of chemo contribute to this blood cancer. My goal is not to create anxiety in those who have received one or more of these drugs, but to raise awareness. Perhaps armed with this information, some may choose to avoid chemotherapy in the future and pursue alternative therapies. Presently, the statistics are: 33 to 55 people are diagnosed with MDS every day (12,000 to 20,000 annually) in the U.S.[32]

It's important to understand that drugs often have more than one name, so please do your research, not only on these drugs, but also on any chemo you may have received or that your oncologist may be recommending. Chemocare[33] is my online go-to resource for information on chemotherapy.

Three of the five chemotherapies Jerry received, cyclophosphamide (Cytoxan®), etoposide (VP-16), and carboplatin, list MDS as a potential side effect.

Other chemotherapies that may also contribute to MDS include:

---

[31] https://www.mds-foundation.org/what-is-mds/
[32] https://www.mds-foundation.org/what-is-mds/
[33] http://chemocare.com/

- chlorambucil
- doxorubicin
- ifosfamide
- mechlorethamine (nitrogen mustard)
- procarbazine
- teniposide

A variety of factors impact the risk of secondary MDS, including the type of chemo and how much is received, in terms of numbers of doses and dosage amounts. Combining radiation with some types of chemo further increases the risk. Unrelated to chemotherapy, but worth mentioning, is that smoking can increase the risk.

So MDS—blood cancer—may be *caused by* chemotherapy and the combination of certain chemotherapies with radiation—the standard cancer treatment protocol! And Jerry had been diagnosed with secondary, or *therapy-related*, MDS.

Unbelievable. His previous chemotherapy treatments had given him cancer four.

Plus, the radiation he received may have been a contributing factor.

I felt angry, but not all that surprised. Jerry's medical records detailing treatment of his first three cancers correlated with the MDS research information.

→ **Etoposide (VP-16):** Here's a quote from earlier in this book: *"Jerry endured three chemo cocktails over the first three days, with two types of chemo, carboplatin and VP-16, in each. The bodily wastes were so toxic that he was told to flush the toilet twice every time he went."* Jerry had received 21 doses of VP-16 during his first cancer, ten years before he developed MDS.

→ **Cyclophosphamide (Cytoxan):** Jerry also had 2 major doses of Cytoxan, for chemo treatments 8 and 9 during his first cancer.

→ **Carboplatin:** Jerry had also been given a total of 23 doses of carboplatin with his first cancer, and 5 doses with radiation during cancer number three (which increases the MDS probability), five years before he developed MDS. (And this leukemia tends to be hard to treat, like the leukemia linked to Cytoxan.)

With his MDS, Jerry had experienced problems with every major facet of his blood: red and white blood cells, platelets, as well as hemoglobin (a component of red blood cells that carries oxygen and nutrients to the cells and collects the carbon dioxide and wastes). I rubbed my eyes and leaned back into the sofa.

Jerry's oncologists had never mentioned cancer as a potential result of treatment, and they'd withheld information that may have influenced the choices we might have made.

Thus, we had been given no choice. The doctors had made the decisions for us.

As I'm writing and reflecting, I wonder. *If* the doctors had let us know that chemotherapy could lead to additional cancer diagnoses, would we have reconsidered? Would we have researched to find out if any choices besides chemotherapy were available?

Jerry's first three cancers had occurred at a time when Internet content was very limited, so we may not have been able to learn of any other options.

A Note about Side Effects of Chemo

Information is often changing, and things above that I found while doing research in 2017 to 2019 might be updated by now. So it's important for you to look up the side effects of the chemo you've received or that your doctor is recommending. Keep in mind that often the brand and generic names differ from each other. Again, I have found Chemocare.com to be a valuable resource.

☐

I couldn't clear my head. The thoughts in it swirled. With phone in hand, I tried to describe my persistent mood to a friend, and cooking terms came to mind. I was stewing, simmering—NO! I was *marinating* in anger, much as Dr. Blinders had marinated my Jerry in chemotherapy. Thankfully, I had a few good friends to share my angst with, because I knew that anger and unforgiveness can be extremely toxic to health.

After talking on the phone, I still needed a break. Often when I needed physical release for troubled emotions, I went out to do yard work or go for a walk. I would also spend a lot of time in prayer, listening to Christian worship music, and experiencing the presence of God to get back into a place of peace. For a few days I tried it all. This time none of it helped.

Writing and researching were taking a toll. At times I couldn't touch the manuscript for days or weeks on end. I found myself grieving, not only for what I discovered in Jerry's medical records, but also because of all that I was learning about the treatment my Jerry had received.

I grieved for people diagnosed with cancer who are still receiving the same chemo and radiation that have been used for—how long? I thought I'd heard "decades" at some point. I found myself questioning when these drugs had come into existence and felt compelled to again search for answers. I can hardly believe what I found.

"The 1943 results set off a burst of support for the synthesis and testing of several related alkylating compounds, including oral derivatives such as chlorambucil and ultimately cyclophosphamide."[34]

"Cyclophosphamide was approved for medical use in the United States in 1959."[35] Jerry had received cyclophosphamide (Cytoxan), and they'd developed it before 1959? With all the horrific side effects that had presented themselves in the decades since then, pharmaceutical companies were still selling it and doctors were still using it? Unbelievable.

Jerry had also received the following three.

"Carboplatin was patented in 1972 and approved for medical use in 1986."[36]

"Etoposide was approved for medical use in the United States in 1983."[37]

"Paclitaxel (PTX), sold under the brand name Taxol . . . was first isolated in 1971 from the Pacific yew and approved for medical use in 1993."[38]

"More than forty years after the war on cancer was declared, we have spent billions fighting the good fight. The National Cancer Institute has spent some $90 billion on research and treatment during that time. Some 260 nonprofit organizations in the United States have dedicated themselves to cancer . . . more than the number established for heart disease, AIDS, Alzheimer's disease, and stroke combined. Together, these 260 organizations have budgets that top $2.2 billion."[39]

It seems scandalous to me that doctors still prescribe these chemo "therapies" to treat cancer, fully understanding that they can and do cause other cancers. It seems scandalous that the FDA allows it. Over all the years, with all

[34] http://cancerres.aacrjournals.org/content/68/21/8643
[35] https://en.wikipedia.org/wiki/Cyclophosphamide
[36] https://en.wikipedia.org/wiki/Carboplatin
[37] https://en.wikipedia.org/wiki/Etoposide
[38] https://en.wikipedia.org/wiki/Paclitaxel
[39] https://www.thedailybeast.com/are-we-wasting-billions-seeking-a-cure-for-cancer

the billions of dollars raised and thrown at cancer research, conventional medicine is still losing the war on cancer.

Eventually my anger subsided. I picked up the file to return to Dr. PM's March 15, 2011, notes.

> PLAN:
> We discussed the bone marrow findings and the serious nature of the marrow dysplasia.
> Treatment is palliative standard therapy would be [   ]. We offered treatment on
> [   ]. He was given a
> consent form and we reviewed both standard treatment and the investigational trial in detail.
> He will consider treatment options and will call us later this week.

from March 15, 2011, document (printout page 75)

In the document section titled "Plan" Dr. PM had written, "We discussed the bone marrow findings and the serious nature of the marrow dysplasia. Treatment is palliative."

Dr. PM hadn't stated the situation in those terms. It was hard to read it now.

"He was given a consent form and we reviewed both standard treatment and the investigational trial in detail. He will consider treatment options and will call us later this week."

"Investigational trial." Often people go through trials in the hope of extending their lives or to contribute to research. We had opted to go search for a better quality of life than we believed the study had offered, firmly believing we would find a cure.

Neither of us ever read the packet that described the study. While sorting the medical records months earlier, I'd set it aside, not believing there would be anything important to include since Jerry hadn't participated in the trial.

But that nagging word *sifting* returned.

I pulled out the packet Dr. PM had given us six years earlier and took a deep breath.

Each time I'd been given the word *sifting* before, I'd discovered something stunning. So, I had reason to anticipate my research now would reveal unexpected news.

Line by line, I read the information about the study cover to cover— nineteen pages of dense, mind-numbing text.

As I read through it a second time to better comprehend it, I read as if Jerry had agreed to participate. The study details became personal.

In short, using a group of about 150 MDS patients, two experimental drugs would be tested, which I'll call drug A and drug B. Volunteer patients in Group A would receive drug A. Volunteer patients in Group B would receive drugs A and B.

The purpose of the study was "to find out what effects, good or bad" the drugs had on the test subjects. On Jerry.

The packet said the drugs could potentially "help" his blood work. But what about the side effects? Incredulously, with *both* drugs, Jerry and the other test subjects could experience *lower* red and white blood cell and platelet counts, plus a host of typical, awful chemotherapy side effects.

In fact, dozens of chemo side effects were listed for each drug—spread over four of the nineteen pages—along with the statement that 10 percent of the subjects "or more" may experience that extent of side effects.

How many more? By lumping those side effects statistics together, I felt there was less accountability. Would some of the side effects impact 25 percent, or 50 percent, or even more of the patients?

My own blood boiled as I kept reading. ". . . We do not know all the effects that may happen." ". . . May be mild or very serious." ". . . Can be life-threatening."

I remembered Dr. PM had said that these experimental drugs "aren't really chemo," and "if there are side effects . . . they will be very mild."

During the study, Jerry would have undergone frequent tests, not the least of which were *several* bone marrow biopsies. It also stated that they'd like additional bone marrow and blood for future research studies, and they'd collect them at the same time while doing the clinical or research collections.

Also, Jerry and the other subjects could volunteer to have two additional bone marrow biopsies, to be used in laboratory studies and/or future research studies.

I shuddered.

Would patients benefit from the drugs? "Taking part . . . may or may not make your health better. . . . There is no proof of this yet. . . . This information could help future cancer patients."

"No proof." "Could."

Dr. PM had told us, "This experimental program is considered the best course of treatment for MDS at this time." How could he have claimed that if the packet to patients hadn't claimed it?

In retrospect, it felt like Jerry had narrowly escaped a potentially dangerous treatment that had been misrepresented by his oncologist, the one person we'd needed to trust with his life.

Suddenly, the packet itself seemed almost ominous.

Would Jerry or any of the test subjects have been compensated? No. The exact wording was, "You will not be paid for being in this study."

Even worse, if Jerry or the others were sick or hurt as a result of being in the trial, they could receive treatment through the doctor/hospital but, "You or your health insurance plan will be billed."

I read on. There were only a few things we wouldn't be billed for. The two voluntary bone marrow biopsies, and the actual drugs that were being studied. If Jerry needed any medications to counteract the side effects, they would be billed to our insurance.

And, believe it or not, the pharmaceutical company wasn't even paying for the study drugs. Those drugs were being funded by The Division of Cancer Treatment and Diagnosis, NCI (National Cancer Institute),[40] and National Institute of Health—government agencies.

Elsewhere in the packet, the study reiterated that the bone marrow and peripheral blood may help to "develop new products" in the future.

Unbelievable. The unspecified entity ordering the drug study, almost certainly a pharmaceutical company, was being paid for the trial drugs by our government. And test subjects were to pay for much of the pharmaceutical company's study. The pharmaceutical company was paying for little of it that I could discern, yet they would end up with new products to sell and profit from?!

Was that why Dr. PM had selected Jerry and encouraged him to participate, because we had good insurance? And if insurance failed to cover it all, Dr. PM believed we could pay for it? I hated to think that had anything to do with it, or that it had everything to do with it, but would Dr. PM have even mentioned the study to us if he knew we couldn't pay to participate?

"You or your health insurance plan will be billed." "Develop new products."

For years I'd known about the pharmaceutical industry, and would cynically talk about the conspiracy, corruption, and collusion between big pharma, the medical community, and our government. While writing I wondered if I should go down this road and include the information in this book. But here it is. Products and profits (billions of dollars) are being generated at the expense of suffering cancer patients, as well as other patients and their families. But, as I read through the experimental study, my outrage was magnified beyond anything I could have imagined. The pages I'd thought would be unimportant actually personified, in my mind, big pharma's desire to use my Jerry as a lab rat, at our expense. And since this is a quest for the truth, I felt compelled to share it with you.

And to keep *sifting*.

☐

---

[40] https://dctd.cancer.gov/default.htm

Wanting recent knowledge and a broad picture of how drug companies operated, I went back to the Internet.

And I immediately found this.

> Imagine an industry that generates higher profit margins than any other and is no stranger to multi-billion dollar fines for malpractice. . . . With some drugs costing upwards of $100,000 for a full course, and with the cost of manufacturing just a tiny fraction of this, it's not hard to see why. . . .
>
> Drug companies justify the high prices they charge by arguing that their research and development (R & D) costs are huge. . . . But . . . drug companies spend far more on marketing drugs—in some cases twice as much—than on developing them. . . .
>
> Drug companies have also been accused of colluding with chemists to overcharge for their medicines and of publishing trial data that highlight the positive at the expense of the negative. . . . The rewards are so great, it would seem, that pharma companies have continually been prepared to push the boundaries of legality. . . .
>
> No wonder, then, that the World Health Organization (WHO) has talked of the "inherent conflict" between the legitimate business goals of the drug companies and the medical and social needs of the wider public.[41]

I lowered my head into my hand, reflecting on that. I had it firsthand, in writing from the experimental study, that cancer patients' insurance companies, and/or the patients themselves, pay to participate in the study, so that drug companies can financially benefit from patients' investments long-term.

My investigative efforts were taking an emotional toll. Exhausted, I fell asleep with the stack of documents and my computer before me. As I awoke, my head snapped back, feeling like I'd given myself whiplash. I couldn't think and threw in the towel for the night. I barely navigated up the stairs to bed.

The next morning, I turned to the last pages of the study packet.

---

[41] http://www.bbc.com/news/business-28212223

Jerry and I were always careful with our personal information, and the study described how Jerry's personal information wouldn't be used, that it would be kept private. It outlined that the study had obtained a Confidentiality Certificate from the Department of Health and Human Services.

On the very next page, however, nine different organizations, government agencies, or businesses were listed who may have access to Jerry's research records, not the least of which were "drug manufacturers and/or their representatives."

What? I went back and studied it. There was only an illusion of confidentiality.

It proceeded to get worse as I read through the Authorization for the Release of Protected Health Information (HIPAA).

First, signing the Personal Health Information (PHI) authorization was mandatory. It included releasing Jerry's medical history and any information collected during the study.

Second, Jerry's PHI could be given to: study sponsors, other investigators (who were they?), regulatory authorities in the U.S. and other countries, and the Institutional Review Board overseeing the study.

Third, it stated plainly, "These records might contain information that identifies you."

The excuse for releasing supposedly confidential information was "to assure the quality of the study, or for other uses allowed by law." Reading that made me extremely uncomfortable.

The next statement had me livid. "Your PHI may no longer be protected under the HIPAA privacy rule once it is given to these other parties." What? Outrageous! It seemed like a complete scam. We're going to protect your identity—maybe? But if we don't, it's fair game?

Is this study typical of other medical studies? I have no idea, but before you agree to participate in a study, I highly recommend reading it thoroughly and taking it to a lawyer. In my mind, carte blanche had been given to the doctors, pharmaceutical companies, governmental agencies, and anyone else who wanted the information—everyone, that is, except the test subjects.

Now, if any of these "experimental study" discoveries up till now has surprised you or made you cautious, hold onto your britches.

A rare but serious side effect that may occur was "Severe reaction of the . . . gut lining that may include . . . shredding or death . . . of tissue."

I now stared at the packet in absolute disbelief.

An MDS patient considering participation would need dogged determination and persistent clarity of mind to get through the dense packet. Anything less, and they'd have to rely on their doctor's assessment of the study, which may or may not be accurately or fully presented.

And of course, the patient selected by the oncologist to participate, but not likely to benefit, would only be chosen if their insurance, or they themselves, could pay for a share of the study.

As I pondered all the nuances of the experimental trial, I could envision Dr. PM rubbing his hands together, anticipating billing for all the appointments, shots, blood work, and everything else he could bill for. He definitely had a financial incentive for recommending the experimental study.

And if Jerry had agreed to participate in the trial, his insurance or our personal money would have contributed to a pharmaceutical business's drug development. It helped to understand that at a personal level, and then expand the scope to consider the impact on society. The outrageous cost of health care that has been crippling so many families and so much of the economy is apparently of little concern to such doctors or big pharma. I wanted to scream.

Were drug companies suffering financially to the extent that they justified guilting cancer patients via oncologists into funding the development of highly profitable drugs?

Why did the world of oncology seem to be more about big money and big pharma, and merely achieving the magical five-year survival rate, than about a cure?

The answer stared up at me from the pages of the experimental drug packet.

Because a genuine cure for cancer, it seemed, would cut deeply into the profits of a multi-billion-dollar industry.[42]

During the hours I'd read through the study packet, anger often arose as I discovered the ugly truth. I almost felt as if Dr. PM had attempted to perpetrate a crime upon us—the deception, fraud, conspiracy, or collusion of the medical system. And this had been yet another oncologist we had trusted to safeguard, above all, my husband's life.

☐

I'll be honest with you, I have become biased, but I believe justifiably so. The more I've researched, the more cynical and outraged I've become. But it

---

[42] https://www.bloomberg.com/news/articles/2019-01-11/big-pharma-faces-the-curse-of-the-billion-dollar-blockbuster

equips me to share. If—God willing—Jerry's and my trials raise awareness, perhaps it'll be worth it all. We became impassioned and wanted to help others, so that no one else should go through what we endured.

Whenever my sifting has uncovered something particularly disturbing, it often took days for me to recover and dig into Jerry's cancer files again. That was the case when my reading the experimental drug study had elevated oncological pharmaceuticals to a whole new level of evil.

As I returned to the manuscript with a fresh resolve, I started researching to corroborate my allegations. Such was the case when I found the article "Spilling the beans—Failure to publish the results of all clinical trials is skewing medical science."

The article reveals that the results of few studies are published, especially if the study does not yield the desired results. The following example is quite an indictment. "In 1994 a study on surgery for bowel cancer found that, among those whose tumors returned, a second visit to the operating theatre to remove the resurgent carcinoma made no difference to life expectancy. Had this information been made public then, rather than as it was in 2014, countless very ill patients could have been spared surgical procedures."[43]

The curtain had been pulled back. A naked block of truth was revealed. There is no reversing that fresh awareness.

Jerry and my desire to write only positives about our cancer journey can't happen, not to the extent we'd wanted it. The truth is more important. More than ever, I am on a quest to unmask, and convey, those truths.

---

[43] https://www.economist.com/science-and-technology/2015/07/25/spilling-the-beans

Chapter 11
Cancer Four: Bone Marrow Treatment

Shortly after the oncology appointment, Jerry and I said no to Dr. PM's standard chemotherapy treatment, and no to the proposed drug study—*"This isn't really chemo,"*—which the doctor had then grudgingly admitted was chemo. That left us at a new crossroads for addressing the MDS, and all options left stood outside the realm of familiar cancer approaches.

Jerry's coworker suggested looking into Dr. Stanislaw Burzynski in Houston, an integrative provider (medical doctor (MD) + holistic). He had been successfully treating cancer with a protocol he himself had invented. We investigated Dr. Burzynski and his treatment, increasingly impressed with his results. However, the treatment was very expensive and, since it was experimental and holistic, probably not covered by insurance.

We kept looking.

A buddy told Jerry about a close friend who'd gone through stem cell (bone marrow) transplant and had success with that. Soon Jerry became optimistic about that option, so his friend connected Jerry with a bone marrow transplant specialist in Chicago.

On March 19, 2011, I completed my education and became a Certified Natural Health Counselor. Personally, I was advocating for natural health modalities to help treat the MDS, but Jerry still had confidence in conventional western medicine. Because of the press, hype, and approval by the insurance companies, he was convinced that the progress of stem cell transplantation offered hope and ultimately a solution. So, it was off to Chicago to start the long process involved with bone marrow treatment.

Every step of the cancer journey seemed to take us further from home. Traveling to Chicago added at least another thirty minutes to our previous hour-plus drive time to chemotherapy, one way. Fortunately, Jerry was back in sales and had a wonderful boss who gave him all the time needed for the doctor appointments and tests. Also, I could arrange my schedule to go with Jerry when he wanted or needed me to go, which was nearly every visit while he was in the bone marrow transplant process.

We moved relatively quickly from Dr. PM to the bone marrow transplant center, only one week between. Jerry continued to have his primary blood work done at Dr. PM's office since it was closer than the bone marrow transplant center—BMTC, to be succinct—and his employer was situated between our home and Dr. PM.

Jerry's medical records had to be forwarded, and many questions needed to be answered before the bone marrow transplant, or BMT, doctor would agree to see him.

In 2011, the restrictions were more stringent on eligibility requirements for a bone marrow transplant than they are today. Jerry was over sixty at the time, so that was a potential issue with the treatment facility. We understood they were looking for candidates whom they felt they could truly help and would not accept anyone with a poor potential for survival. (At least that was what we were told.)

I, like so many others, felt confused about the difference between bone marrow transplant and stem cell transplant. Bone marrow transplant was the term we'd heard most often, and that was what we used in our CaringBridge posts, so for consistency and brevity BMT is what I've continued to use. But the process and terminology have evolved, so I thought the following overview might help.

> In the past, patients who needed a stem cell transplant received a "bone marrow transplant" because the stem cells were collected from the bone marrow. Today, stem cells are usually collected from the blood, instead of the bone marrow. So now they are more commonly called stem cell transplants.[44]

Our first appointment with the BMT coordinator and doctor was in late March. Before meeting the doctor, Jerry/we had mountains of paperwork to work through—insurance and financial documents, a durable power of attorney for health care, medical release authorization, pages upon pages of information about the bone marrow transplant program, and patient demographics. Nurse Tanya went through all the paperwork with us. Jerry was hopeful and optimistic, and I was supportive. Looking at all the paperwork, it felt like we were signing his life away.

After the paperwork had been completed, the bone marrow transplant doctor met with us. He explained the process and procedures of looking for a donor. First, they would send a kit to family members. Jerry had a brother, John. If he

---

[44] http://www.cancer.net/navigating-cancer-care/how-cancer-treated/bone-marrowstem-cell-transplantation/what-stem-cell-transplant-bone-marrow-transplant

was a close match, we'd be thankful and lucky. If not, then the BMTC would start searching for a match. The donors are not limited to a certain geographic area. They can search worldwide.

Of course, the doctor and staff were positive and upbeat, convincing us that this was Jerry's/our best hope.

I kept asking questions about natural health and building up Jerry's immune system prior to the actual bone marrow transplant. "Dr. BMT" kept responding that they would have to review everything before Jerry could use any supplements, and that he could use nothing but what the transplant team approved of after the transplant.

At home, I suggested to Jerry that we consistently eat healthier foods while waiting for the bone marrow transplant, and again recommended the Budwig Diet, to improve his immune system.

His response? "They're going to kill my immune system anyway, so what's the point?"

We have to choose our battles, and this wasn't something we needed to battle over. He needed my support, so I threw my love and support his way. I really had to suck it up and concede, which wasn't easy, knowing all that I knew about healing from the inside out.

⬜

Jerry felt thankful when the bone marrow transplant center accepted him into the program. That set our course for the next three months.

Our children drove up from Texas together in early April. When they arrived, we had serious talks about the diagnosis and options available, and the decisions that we'd made and why. With all that out of the way, we took a few days to have fun.

One day my parents drove out, and we spent it at the Volo Auto Museum that has hundreds of collector cars. My dad had lots of car stories, and of course Jerry was always a car guy. We all found favorites, from antique models my dad had once driven, to cars from movies, including the Ecto-1 Ghostbusters Car and the DeLorean from *Back to the Future*, Devin's favorite.

We laughed and reminisced, and life was good. And normal.

Since we'd moved six times with our children, my parent's home of more than fifty years remained one of their favorite places to be. It's decorated with love and holds our family's history, with all the treasures in the same places. We are reminded of gifts given, stories told, games played, puzzles put together, and most of all, the endless hours of entertainment at the foosball table. It's wonderful to be able to return to a place with so much love and peace during stressful times.

Back at our own house, Jerry, the kids, and I took one day to finish some landscaping projects, including a landscaping wall, knowing that the months ahead would be filled with challenges. That night, after dinner, we pulled out the storage bins that held the kids' childhood keepsakes. What great memories! Gymnastics memorabilia, baseball cards, soccer stuff, trophies, medals, photographs, and favorite toys were just some of the items in those treasure troves of special times.

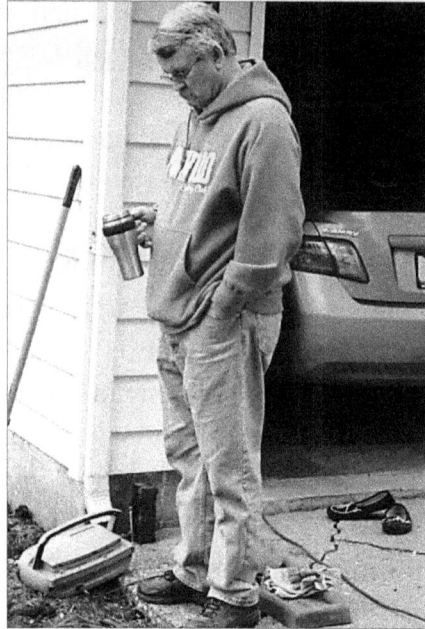

My fondest memory of the kids' visit was when each of them put on one of their favorite shirts from their youth. Brandon donned his St. Louis Cardinals jersey that he'd worn when he was about eleven years old. Devin was able to get into his gymnastics uniform shirt he'd competed in at age nine, and Tara squeezed into the gymnastics T-shirt she'd gotten for Christmas when she was five. They all had a lot of trouble trying to wriggle out of the shirts, and almost had to be cut out of them.

Jerry and I had raised wonderfully funny and slightly nutty kids. Thankfully, they were all strong and resilient in the face of Jerry's cancer diagnosis. We felt incredible pride in them.

It was hard to watch them pile into the truck to head back to Texas, but we'd had a lot of fun, and had faced reality. It helped Brandon, Devin, and Tara to see that Jerry and I stood united and hopeful about the future, as always. And we knew that our strength and courage had been passed on to our children as they returned to their homes and lives 1200 miles away.

☐

Jerry had remained resilient throughout all his cancer odysseys, but he was about to become much more so during this next trial.

Though generally a private person, Jerry opted to make his cancer journey public as he started the BMT process. He began posting on www.CaringBridge.org on April 15, 2011, less than three months after being diagnosed with MDS. CaringBridge is a free blogsite for people experiencing serious illness or difficult pregnancies. Jerry knew it would be helpful to keep our friends and family on the same page so that we wouldn't get overwhelmed with phone calls, e-mails, and repeating the same information over and over.

How it worked was simple. Every time we posted a journal entry at CaringBridge, those who'd signed up to be notified would receive an e-mail. They, in turn, could stay current by reading our updates, and post prayers, comments, and words of encouragement.

Jerry and I found the process of writing the journal very therapeutic and helpful in the journey, and I highly recommend this fabulous resource for anyone going through a difficult health issue. (The collection of blog posts served as the basis for the original draft of this book.)

A Note about Our CaringBridge Posts

Parts of our journey that were documented at CaringBridge are sprinkled over the pages ahead, positive attitudes and good humor intact. Our posts from that site appear in *italics*, edited only for logical readability, to remove redundancies, and alter names for privacy. The essence has not changed.

When we started the blog, Jerry said, "I want to keep everything positive. Let's not write anything that will cause our family or friends to worry. We'll put off posting until we can put a positive spin on it." So that's what we did.

If we titled a post, it's been included here.

Often, I ended my posts with the words *In Christ* or *In Him*, or a similar expression of the faith that carried us through, but the repetitiveness seemed to detract rather than add to the reading. So, I have not included them.

My comments, reflections, and other nuggets that I've added for clarity or understanding, appear in regular font.

One of the main reasons I wanted to write about Jerry's cancer journey was to share the positive attitude we carried throughout. (Choose your attitude, and make it a good one! One of the four pillars.) You may not be able to control all that is happening in your life, but you *can* choose your attitude!

Journal entry by JERRY HUSSEY—4/15/2011

    We found out Monday that my brother is not a good match to use his stem cells in my bone marrow transplant. He matched just three of the six markers.

    Shortly after learning that my brother was not a match, I received a call from Nurse Tanya advising me that they had found a preliminary match from the donor list. An individual had registered with a donor program somewhere in the world. The BMTC has to contact that donor program and have them contact the donor. If the donor is still around and is still willing to donate, a sample of his/her blood will be sent to the BMTC for further matching. If that is a good match, we get the donor to Chicago, to the BMTC, and conduct actual bone barrow comparisons. This whole process with an unknown donor takes about three months.

    I go to my regular oncologist/hematologist on Monday 4/17 for blood labs to see where my platelets are. If they are too low, I will get a transfusion of platelets and continue doing my job. We will post more when we know about my platelet count and any updates on a donor.

    Thanks for tagging along.

Journal entry by JERRY HUSSEY—4/19/2011

    I do believe God is watching over us. I received an e-mail from the transplant coordinator that the donor that had been identified is still in the program and has submitted a blood sample. It will take about one and a half to two weeks to determine the suitability. If that match comes through, the next step is to get the donor to Chicago to undergo a bone marrow sampling to compare with mine.

    Keep praying, my friends and family, and while you pray, please include my boss's husband, Rich, the pancreatic cancer fighter.

Moving Right Along—Journal entry by JERRY HUSSEY—5/18/2011

    Nurse Tanya called today saying the donor has agreed to come to Chicago and continue the process. All I know is that it is a he, and he is thirty-two years old.

    Late next week, or possibly the following week, I have to go to the bone marrow transplant center to begin qualifying to make sure all of my systems and functions are strong enough to handle this. It kind of reminds me of Arlo Guthrie at the induction center in the song "Alice's Restaurant."

The testing will take at least two full days and possibly a third for both of us. Once the tests are completed and evaluated, with all systems a go, then we begin the transplant procedure.

The fact that we are getting closer to the transplant is both exciting and a little scary. Please continue your thoughts and prayers for me, as I do appreciate them.

God bless you all!

Now We Are in High Gear!—*Journal entry by* JERRY HUSSEY—*5/19/2011*

Between now and June 15, I will have four trips to the bone marrow transplant center for tests and checkups. I will get the alphabet soup of tests: EEG, EKG, CT, and whatever else they think of. I will be fitted with a port and will have that evaluated a couple of times to make sure it works right before they kill my immune system.

I have blood work 5/23 and 6/8 at Dr. PM's office to determine if I need another transfusion. May 25 I have a long day of labs at the BMTC.

June 2, 7, and 9 @ the BMTC—additional testing, bone marrow biopsy, and final CT scan before beginning chemo.

My beloved donor will be going through the same procedures, except for the port. Bone marrow collection to start 6/20 and take two days.

Admission date scheduled for 6/15 with chemotherapy to kill my bone marrow. My bone marrow transplant will begin on 6/21 or 6/22 and last about one and a half to two hours.

Barring rejection and any complications, I should be released around 8/1 (FYI: The doctor and bone marrow transplant team estimated Jerry would be in the hospital up to six weeks!) *but will have to go back to the hospital twice weekly for checkups for six months following discharge.*

This is all tentative. . . .

Please continue your thoughts and prayers that I will make it through this ordeal, and please, please continue praying for my friend Rich, who is having a lot of difficulties with his medical staff.

God bless you all!

One More Blood Test—Journal entry by JERRY HUSSEY—5/23/2011

Today I had to go to the oncologist's office to let them take more of my blood for evaluation. . . . My platelets dropped 1000 from the last check, and my hemoglobin increased just a bit. According to the BMTC that's a good sign that I will not have to have another transfusion before the transplant.

I also received my written itinerary for the next three weeks of testing at the bone marrow transplant center. There may be a problem—I have to have a psychological evaluation! Does that mean I'll have to go to the Group W bench? (From the song "Alice's Restaurant." We were told that the psychological exam was one of the most important exams. The stress of going through the whole process before, during, and after the transplant was arduous, and the BMTC would not take anyone they thought couldn't complete it. Four to six weeks in the hospital for the transplant and recovery alone was enough to break some. Again, "Alice's Restaurant." ☺)

The lab report on May 24 compared the donor's blood markers with Jerry's. They were amazingly similar—5 of 6 markers matched perfectly!

As ET Would Say, "Oooouuuch"—Journal entry by JERRY HUSSEY—5/25/2011

Actually, the tests went well, and I'm glad to know my heart is healthy and beating the way it is supposed to beat. I had an EKG, and all of my valves and other functions are completely normal. . . .

On the bad side, one component of my blood is critically low, but there is nothing that can be done except be very, verrrrrry careful. It is a component that activates immune function, and it is so low I can eat no raw foods— protein, fruits, or vegetables—except thick-skinned fruits like bananas and watermelon. I cannot be around crowds, and I am supposed to wear a mask if someone in the office or here at home is sick. If I get a fever over 100.6, I am supposed to rush to the closest emergency room and have antibiotics injected.

Finally, I had the bone marrow draw for biopsy. <u>Don't ever let anyone tell you that it is not painful.</u> Even with a local anesthetic I felt most of what was going on, and when the needle broke through the bone to get to the marrow, I almost wet my pants. Then, they had to go feeling around with the slip joint pliers to find the most painful spot to break off a piece of hipbone to *be biopsied. Unfortunately, I have to undergo many more of these procedures, and I do hope my hip bone regenerates.*

(Remember that the donor was going through this same procedure. I think anyone who goes through this for a complete stranger, or even someone they know, deserves to be called a hero and should get some kind of award. Even today my heartfelt thanks goes out to the young man who endured a bone marrow biopsy to try to help Jerry. It is a shame that most of these donations are anonymous and we never get to thank the person who went over and above to try to give someone their life back. I hope he reads this book, recognizes himself, and gets in touch via my website.)[45]

After all that, Diane and I spent about an hour with Nurse Tanya discussing the procedures and expected side effects of the drugs they will be giving me. Once I am out of the hospital, I will have to go back twice weekly for six months or more to monitor the antirejection drugs I will be on. . . .

While I'm a patient in the hospital . . . I will require a mask and gloves when I go outside my room. I can have any healthy guests . . . but the guests will be gowned, masked, and gloved.

There is a cot available, and Diane can stay overnight if we so desire. Diane can bring outside food in, as long as the food isn't raw and is approved.

After the transplant and during my hospital stay, I will need lots of platelets. Nurse Tanya asked us to contact friends and relatives to ask that you donate platelets on my behalf. . . .

(Remember, I donated platelets when we lived in San Antonio. Things always seem to come back full circle.)

The target date is still June 15 for admittance to the hospital. . . . It is a blessing to know the rest of my body is in good shape so far, and I think we will find the rest of the testing to be a breeze.

Please continue prayers for me, and please keep Rich in your prayers also. It seems he has received a good break lately, so your prayers are working.

God bless you all.

---

[45] www.dianebishophussey.com

On June 2, 2011, Jerry and I went to his regularly scheduled BMTC appointment. He had just taken the psychological test, and the related BMTC report was complete. According to the bone marrow transplant center's psychologist, our doctor said, Jerry was mentally and emotionally sound to undergo the transplant.

Right there in the BMTC office, I beamed to hear that, proud of Jerry and his positive mindset despite his health challenges.

A Note about Stem Cell Transplantation

To provide some clarity, the first part of the stem cell transplant process is called *conditioning*. During this time, Jerry would receive chemotherapy and/or radiation to damage and possibly destroy his bone marrow.

The stem cell transplant itself replaces the damaged bone marrow with healthy stem cells. Think of stem cell transplantation as a transfusion of blood and immune cells rather than a surgical procedure.[46]

During the appointment, while Jerry and I consulted with the BMT team and doctor, Jerry pressed a hand to his chest and leaned forward a little.

He said, "Doc, my heart rate has been 150 plus for the previous two mornings." He shook his head, as if confused about it. "And I feel extremely fatigued."

I stared at him. Why didn't he call the doctor to report this? And why didn't he tell me? Denial and desperation for the transplant? Not wanting anything to jeopardize it?

Dr. BMT was already on his feet and closing the distance between his stethoscope and Jerry. He listened to Jerry's heart, his face showing concern, and then alarm.

He glanced at the nearest member of his team. "Get a tech with a gurney up here, *STAT*!"

The team member ran out the door.

I stood up, cold apprehension crawling over my skin. *What was happening?*

The team cleared to the sides of the small room just as the door burst open with a tech and two nurses bringing in a gurney. Rapidly they helped Jerry onto it.

---

[46] https://www.dana-farber.org/health-library/articles/what-happens-during-the-stem-cell-transplant-process-/

Moments later the tech was pushing Jerry on the gurney, the two nurses and me flying along beside them, taking back hallways, rushing from the doctor's office in the tower down to the ED—Emergency Department.

Eight days ago, Jerry's heart had been just fine. Why the change? Why now? Was God trying to tell us something?

Soon I was standing in the ED looking down at Jerry. He'd just had a CT scan and a chest x-ray. Now he was hooked up with more wires than an electronic experiment.

So far all we knew was that he didn't have a pulmonary embolism (blood clot) or pneumonia. His heart rate was still high.

The ED doctor appeared again. "Jerry, we're going to admit you to the hospital to keep an eye on you. We should have answers in the morning."

I took hold of Jerry's hand, my thoughts spiraling, but held myself together. I stayed with Jerry and stayed positive.

He was admitted to a room late in the day, looking exhausted. After a kiss and a prayer together, I headed home. I had to get back to let the dog out, or else I'd have stayed with Jerry, as well as avoided the hour-and-a-half drive.

Before I could go to sleep, I needed to update our friends and family through CaringBridge. *Keep it positive*, I reminded myself, and then started typing.

Speed Bump—Journal entry by DIANE HUSSEY—6/2/2011

Don't you just hate it when you're flying along and hit a speed bump? Or you're making really good time and have to slow down for one of those doggone things?

That's how we felt today. Jerry went in for a couple of tests (he didn't even study for them but passed with flying colors!). He did the pulmonary (lung) and psychology tests.

But his heart was beating too fast and he had an irregular heartbeat, so they tried to determine the cause. For starters, a CT scan to rule out a blood clot in the lungs.

Praise God—no blood clot! But they don't know what is causing the rapid heartbeat, so they decided to keep him overnight for observation.

More later—it's been a LONGGGG day.

The next day was a long one as well.

When I arrived, Jerry wasn't in his room. I was told that Jerry's symptoms were due to atrial fibrillation—a-fib—an irregular heartbeat. Essentially, the electrical signals controlling his heart's rhythm were out of whack. A surgical team was performing a cardiac ablation to get it back into rhythm.

Hours passed before Jerry was finally rolled back into his room. He gave me a tired smile but looked better than he had.

Late that night and for the following few nights, I kept friends and family apprised of Jerry's updates through our CaringBridge blog.

The Way to a Man's Heart—Journal entry by DIANE HUSSEY—6/3/2011

They say the way to a man's heart is through his stomach. That's close— it's through his groin.

Today Jerry had two procedures. They rammed a tube down his throat so they could do an ultrasound on his heart to make sure he had no blood clots in there.

Then they did an ablation—ran a blowtorch from his groin to his heart to fry the defective circuit in his ventricle so that it would stop fluttering.

So, I missed seeing Jerry before he went into surgery by less than five minutes (nearly two hours to get here) and he didn't get back until about 6:00. He is doing just fine. I'm here next to his bed typing while he's on the phone. He should be able to get up and start dancing by 10:00 p.m.

The main concern, of course, is the timing of all this in relation to the bone marrow transplant. The heart doctor just came in to say Jerry might be able to go home tomorrow if they can get approval from the bone marrow transplant team and if they come into agreement on blood thinner meds.

We are very hopeful, and the doctors think the bone marrow transplant can continue on schedule.

Training Camp Complete—Journal entry by DIANE HUSSEY—6/4/2011

Let's just consider the past few days as a training camp in preparation for the real adventure. Jerry is certainly happy to be home again, and the dog is happy to see him as well.

The doctors must think Jerry's part vampire. They gave him another unit of blood. That's three pints in the past month. They weren't sure why his hemoglobin went down so quickly. Well, DUH—they're always coming in and drawing a few more vials.

All in all, a pretty good trial run. The nurses were great, and the staff was caring and considerate. I guess the bone marrow transplant center passed the test and Jerry will go back for more.

Home for the Moment—Journal entry by JERRY HUSSEY—6/5/2011

It is good to be home, having come through this episode without disrupting the bone marrow transplant. My transplant specialist seems to think we are still on schedule and he will be able to deal with the blood thinners I have to take for four weeks to keep a clot from forming in my heart.

I am overwhelmed at the love, care, and prayers on my behalf. It is great to have wonderful family and friends, and I seem to be overly blessed. Thank you all and continue your thoughts and prayers. The battle has yet to begin!

God bless you all!

On June 7, Jerry went through another CT scan of the chest, plus a CT of his abdomen and pelvis, an ultrasound of the upper arms and chest for placement of the port, and then a doctor appointment to meet the surgeon who was to install the port.

At the appointment, the surgeon got into a dither over the low numbers of Jerry's hemoglobin and platelets. (We'll call the surgeon Dr. Port, for obvious reasons.)

He took one look at Jerry's blood work and asked us, "What's the plan? I need the platelets to be at 50K, and I can't install a port with his hemoglobin this low. What do they expect me to do with these numbers? I need a plan! I need a plan!"

That was the condensed version of probably a two-minute tirade about "the plan." He left the room and came back about five minutes later, still muttering about "the plan."

Jerry and I were mostly doing whatever the doctors said, and we knew Dr. Port had to talk to the other doctors to figure out the hemoglobin. It wouldn't have mattered a lick if we knew what "the plan" was.

On the way home, we reflected on the appointment—"I need a plan!"—and burst into laughter. At least the surgeon had provided some comic relief to a very busy and stressful day!

☐

June 9, 2011, fell on a Thursday. Our hopes fell this day also.

During our appointment with Dr. BMT and the transplant team, the doctor shared some news.

"Jerry, the CT scan showed a suspicious spot in the upper left lobe of your lung that has started to grow. We'll need to do a PET scan to see whether it is cancer."

Jerry and I went still as the implications sank in.

My Jerry currently had blood cancer, and now a new lung nodule? If the nodule proved to be cancer, it would be his fifth.

And the bone marrow transplant would never take place.

The doctor and team waited quietly nearby while Jerry and I absorbed what he'd said. His words repeated themselves in my mind, over and over, until all words fell away except four: *"has started to grow."*

That meant they had been aware of the lung nodule. How long had they known about it?

Jerry and I had never been informed of it until now.

The news struck me with the trauma of being hit by an out-of-control cement truck.

Again the doctor said that Jerry needed a PET scan. He added, "Jerry, the bone marrow transplant will be postponed until the scan results are in."

I'm not sure Jerry or I heard much beyond that. We were too devastated to find that all that we had pinned our hopes on had come crashing down.

We left the office, neither of us talking much.

The CaringBridge blog would sit quiet this night. But Jerry journaled the next day, Friday evening.

Journal entry by JERRY HUSSEY—6/10/2011
As we left the hospital late yesterday afternoon (Thursday) after yet another day of checkups, comparisons, and lab work, Diane and I were almost in tears and at wits' end. The doctor informed us that a nodule in my lung, which had apparently been visible via CT scan for quite a while, has

suddenly decided to grow. Until it is determined what this nodule is, the bone marrow procedure has been postponed. A PET scan is needed to determine if the nodule is active cancer or inflammation from my illness.

All of the above was Satan's way of getting us away from God and His healing power. If you believe, you will understand what I am saying a little bit further along in this missive.

After unloading my angst on my dear Kris, my boss who is the wife of Rich, who is also battling cancer, Diane and I decided to try a different way home. (Thank you, Kris, for your shoulder. You mean a lot to me.)

Anyway, after fighting rush hour traffic, and with the time approaching 6:30 p.m., we decided to stop for dinner at a restaurant we'd never tried before.

Here is where God began working His miracles!

After we received our food and began to eat, a minister we know came over and said hi. He and his wife had chosen that restaurant also. This minister is a preacher of the Bible, God's Word, and does not hold back. After Diane and I ate, we joined them and discussed a bit of our day. I told him my cancer was back, but he would not accept that it is "my" cancer. He said Satan was trying to take me away from God. The four of us joined in prayer there at the table. This minister is a true prayer warrior, and he prayed for Jesus to step in and take over my life.

Diane and I came away from the restaurant and the impromptu prayer meeting with a much lighter step and a more positive attitude.

We had chosen to go home from the hospital a different way than normal. Was God directing us? I think so.

We had stopped at a restaurant that neither of us were familiar with and found a minister we knew there. Did God cause this to happen? I think so.

This morning I received two or three calls from the bone marrow transplant nurse saying, first of all, that she is pushing every power that be, to get financing approved for the PET scan. By 9:30 a.m., I had a call from the PET scan technician saying he could get me in Tuesday at noon, and we made the appointment.

I should probably explain that it takes twenty-four hours to read a PET scan, and I cannot be admitted for the bone marrow transplant prior to the PET scan being read. Even if the nodule is benign, a Tuesday PET scan would make it the following Friday or Monday before I could be admitted and begin the BMT.

After dinner Diane and I checked our phones when we got in the car.

Shirley, my temporary bone marrow transplant nurse, had left a message. I called her back. We talked about the impromptu prayer meeting (she is a devoted Christian, by the way), and I told her of my appointment on Tuesday for the PET scan. Shirley decided that wasn't quick enough. She made a few calls and managed to get me rescheduled for a PET scan on Monday morning at 9:00. And, she used her bully pulpit to get a quick reading so my bone marrow transplant may not be delayed, or at least be delayed as much.

This was about 7:30 p.m. tonight. Why was this nurse still on duty, and why did she get involved this evening? I think God told her that I needed a little help, and could she get involved.

Tanya, my normal bone marrow transplant nurse, is on vacation this week. Did God put Shirley in touch with us to take over the reins, give us support and peace, and take up our battles? I think so.

Within two miles of leaving the restaurant, Thursday evening, I received a vision. It was Peter, walking on water, as long as he kept his eyes on Jesus. The instant he was distracted by the wind and the waves, he started sinking (Matthew 14:28-31). During the drive home, I mentioned the vision to Jerry, and said, "As long as we keep our eyes on Jesus, we'll be okay. We won't sink."

Jerry agreed.

☐

We both resolved to keep that image at the forefront of our minds, and often found ourselves clinging to that image from that day forward.

It seems appropriate to briefly talk about the evolution of our faith here, since between the restaurant and the evening phone calls with the nurse, Jerry had just had a serious "come-to-Jesus" moment. Jerry had never talked much about his faith, God, or attended church regularly as an adult. He'd been raised in the church and was always comfortable with his relationship with God, but on weekends he just wanted to relax at home and catch up on projects or other things he couldn't do while on the road.

On the other hand, I had developed a deep thirst for knowing God more closely. I often sought Him, not only through regular church attendance and Bible studies, but through many other avenues. I had been growing in my personal relationship with Jesus, which was great for me, but it hadn't been bringing Jerry and me closer together.

It's almost funny—I felt like I was chasing God, and God was chasing Jerry. This night at the restaurant, and during the days that followed, it was as if God had reached down and grabbed Jerry, brought him close, and had a heart-to-heart. God had touched him, and Jerry began changing in a huge way.

Like Jerry explained, *"This minister is a true prayer warrior, and he prayed for Jesus to step in and take over my life."* God did exactly that.

Both Jerry and I understood that we needed to keep our eyes on Jesus, and that He would lead us to a faith, trust, and belief strong enough to carry us through anything.

Our Savior would keep Himself, Jerry, and me bound together like a three-strand cord. Two are stronger than one, and when you bring Christ into the equation, "A cord of three strands is not easily broken" (Ecclesiastes 4:12 CSB) and, "With God all things are possible" (Matthew 19:26 CSB).

Before Jerry's come-to-Jesus moment, he'd wrapped up many of his blog posts with requests for prayer. A few hours after that experience, he no longer saw the good events in his days as simple happenstance, but as God's constant presence and immeasurable love.

This is how he ended that Friday evening's blog post.

Journal entry by JERRY HUSSEY—6/10/2011, continued

One of my customers told me that God was going to cure me and that I should believe that because a donor was found so quickly. I firmly believe that, and I believe God has His hand on my shoulder, directing Diane and me down the proper path. Satan is doing all he can to sidetrack this road to a cure, but he can take all of his efforts and stick them in his pointy little ears. WE ARE NOT PARTICIPATING IN HIS ENDEAVORS!

Thank You, my Lord, for taking care of the heart problem without disrupting the bone marrow transplant at that time. Continue Your care and guidance, and we can get through the rest of these obstacles and continue our focus on You.

Friends, today has been a most prayerful day for me, giving thanks to God for the chance meeting with the minister, the scheduling and then rescheduling the PET scan, and prayer that the nodule be directed by Him. It is His will, not my will. Diane and I are at peace, but we are rejoicing in our life and we just keep on smiling!

We promised ourselves that we would post nothing negative on this site unless we could make it fun. As you know, we didn't post last night because most all we had was negative and God had not worked His miracle yet. This miracle that God keeps on working is more powerful than our positive attitudes and our frivolity to make our friends and family comfortable with what is going on. We are experiencing God's work, firsthand.

If all of my talk about God and miracles makes you uncomfortable, maybe you should reexamine your relationship with God. If you are not following in God's footsteps, maybe your life would be a whole lot better if you would. God will test you to the nth degree, but He is a forgiving God and will forgive you if you ask.

Thank you for your prayers and support, and thank You, Lord, for putting this conversation on my chest. I pray it has effect.

That weekend, while Jerry and I waited for his Monday PET scan appointment to come, we discussed probability and options out in Jerry's breezy, sunlit garage. With a bottomless passion for working on his '65 Mustang, and an equally bottomless cup of coffee, Jerry spent as much time in the garage as in the house, the overhead door open, the smell of chrome polish and wax in the air.

I leaned against the door of the car. "Jerry, if this lung nodule turns out to be cancer, what do you think the next move should be?" I held up a hand. "Before you say, 'more chemo,' I have to tell you that I don't believe the medical industry wants a cure for cancer."

He glanced up from under the hood, his skepticism apparent. "Diane, you're crazy."

"Actually, I'm not. There's too much money in cancer. You know that documentary I recently watched, *Burzynski: Cancer Is Serious Business*? It's about Dr. Stanislaw Burzynski, the alternative medicine practitioner who discovered a cure for cancer years ago. His patients and their families overwhelmingly declare he has a cure, though the FDA and others who profit from cancer have been taking him to court for years."

"Has he been found guilty of anything?"

"Not one thing."

Jerry's expression shifted to one of consideration.

That night he and I watched the movie.

Within the first five minutes of the documentary, Jerry was outraged. After the movie, he hopped on the Internet and started researching. He no longer thought I was crazy. The documentary changed everything he had previously thought about the cancer industry, or as I fondly say, "Jerry turned on a dime and gave nine cents change."

If you feel doubtful, I challenge you to watch not only the documentary[47] (it's had more than 930,000 views, as of this writing), but also additional videos regarding Dr. Burzynski's trials that have been posted since 2011. Due to the persecution and prosecution, he has had to move his practice to Mexico, as others have.

☐

On Monday morning, June 13, Jerry went for his nine o'clock PET scan. As Nurse Shirley had promised, the PET scan was read soon after. That same day, the results were faxed to us.

The lung nodule proved to be malignant, Jerry's fifth cancer. The bone marrow transplant was cancelled.

Journal entry by DIANE HUSSEY—6/13/2011

Have you ever started a journey and knew where you wanted to go, but just weren't quite sure how to get there? Sometimes you take the fastest, most direct route, and sometimes you take the scenic route. Sometimes your best plan is sidetracked due to a detour.

It seems we continue to find the detours. Last week they saw something on the CT scan that concerned them, so today they did a PET scan. It kind of sounds like we're going to a vet, doesn't it?

So, time for a new course. There are many alternatives to consider. Jerry will need a biopsy to determine the exact kind of lung cancer so an appropriate course of treatment can be established.

We are not ruling out anything at this time, including alternative cancer therapies. We are also considering going to Houston to see Dr. Burzynski,[48] who found a cure for cancer more than thirty years ago.

---

[47] *Burzynski: Cancer Is Serious Business:* https://www.youtube.com/watch?v=rBUGVkmmwbk
[48] Dr. Burzynski has had to move his operation to Mexico due to the harassment and baseless lawsuits brought against him.

> *Dr. Burzynski's information and video,* Burzynski: Cancer Is Serious Business, *seriously cracked Jerry's faith in American cancer treatments. It exposes the conspiracy, corruption, and collusion between the FDA, big pharma, National Cancer Institute, the doctors, medical boards, and others.*
>
> *We both encourage you to watch this exposé. It is a scathing indictment of an agenda focused on destroying an individual who actually found a cure for cancer.*
>
> *We still have the faith that will move mountains. We have a strong and mighty God who can choose to heal through His healing touch.*
>
> *God's greatest miracle is our human body, which has the ability to heal itself if we give it what it needs. Please stand with us in prayer because we see Jerry's healing as a testimony of our loving God's faithfulness.*

☐

I had suggested to Jerry that we implement some natural health protocols while waiting for the bone marrow transplant and had suggested the Budwig Diet to improve his immune system. His response was along the lines that they were going to kill his immune system anyway, so what's the point?

Here's my take. We fight the battle with cancer, and fight any battle, on four levels—physical, mind (mental/emotional), financial, and spiritual. Where were Jerry and I in the battle? Let's look at the physical aspect in an analogy.

Think of an athlete with a knee injury. Now compare that athlete to someone who never exercises. If both were to require the same exact surgery, and everything was equal in terms of the surgeon and rehab, who do you think would have the best odds of the quickest, most complete healing?

The athlete wants to get back in the game and is motivated to work hard to do so. Athletes are also stronger physically, so doing rehab is not nearly as difficult. To put it into perspective with Jerry, he couldn't understand the merit in being strong physically going into the stem cell treatment. What do you think the odds were in that situation?

Financially, Jerry had excellent insurance, and although we weren't rich, we had resources, so the financial aspect wasn't as daunting as it may be for some. Natural health has many options that are far more reasonably priced than conventional treatments and not nearly as debilitating.

But what about the spiritual battle? Some people feel it's foolish to believe in God's healing over trusting man and man's science. But if you research people's experiences with miraculous healing, or healing through items in nature that God created, you may be surprised to find your own faith getting kicked up a notch. God has blessed many physicians and scientists to make discoveries that heal, so it's important to be well-informed to help you balance science, nature, and faith. That knowledge and balance brings hope.

Thankfully, God brought Jerry and me to the same place through entirely different routes, as I explained earlier. I had actively sought out a personal relationship with Jesus Christ for years. Although Jerry was a believer, and knew *of* God, he didn't really *know* God until he'd experienced the serious come-to-Jesus moment, which happened shortly after we learned about the nodule in his lung that cancelled the bone marrow transplant. Through that event God transformed Jerry and brought him to the next level—an amazingly intimate and personal relationship.

Now, finally, Jerry and I were on the same page. We had the same playbook. And not only were we in lockstep on the health treatment plan, as you're about to see, we'd also arrived on the same spiritual plane.

☐

Three days after I'd typed my last CaringBridge entry, my fingers rattled off the next one. A lot had happened, fast.

Journal entry by D*IANE* H*USSEY*—*6/16/2011*

It's hard to believe it was just Monday that they found lung cancer and determined Jerry is no longer a candidate for the stem cell transplant.

It's equally hard to believe that June 15, the targeted date for admission for the stem cell process to begin, came and went uneventfully yesterday after we'd waited so long.

This morning he was scheduled for a biopsy to determine the course of treatment. We were both in kind of a funk on the way to the hospital.

When the tech who was supposed to do the biopsy came in, it really seemed like he didn't want to do the procedure. "Um, the nodule is, um really small, um close to two blood vessels, um could collapse the lung." He gave all kinds of excuses.

Jerry asked him if he was confident he could do the procedure. We've never heard a weaker, more unsure response. I asked how many of these procedures he'd done. His response? "Um, probably, um hundreds, um maybe two a week, um—" We walked out. Neither one of us had ANY confidence in him.

Then off to Dr. PM's office. Jerry had blood drawn. It continues to remain amazingly stable.

We started talking on the way home, and everything seemed to take us further and further from conventional medical treatment. It is amazing how different our attitudes were from our drive to the hospital, to our drive home.

After we got home, we researched various alternative treatment therapies, and Jerry found one that he is confident and optimistic about. I am in complete agreement, so it appears that Jerry has closed the door on conventional medicine and is now looking at alternative medicine for his CURE!!!! He sent an e-mail to the clinic, and we hope to talk to them tomorrow about starting treatment. We will let you know more details as we confirm them.

We are optimistic and excited to be making the changes in our lives and diets that WILL cure him by building his immune system, instead of poisoning it! Thanks everyone for your prayers! They are working, and we are embarking on a new journey! It's not called survival, it's called LIFE!!!!

We continue to thank God for His blessings and look forward to hearing the miraculous words, "You're cured!"

Please pray for Jerry's brother, John, who is in the hospital with gallstones/gallbladder infection and an arrhythmia.

Please also pray for our friend, Rich, who is traveling to the Burzynski Clinic in Houston for his treatment.

So, we were starting down a whole new path, having closed the door on prior treatment options. In hindsight I think it helpful that the technician had been inept. It made it so easy for Jerry to walk out and not look back.

He now felt as eager as me to pursue an option other than conventional medicine to get to the bottom of his cancer.

Finally, we were on the same page all around.

The next day Jerry plunked down in front of the keyboard.

Glow-in-the-Dark—Journal entry by JERRY HUSSEY—6/17/2011
I have been going through my records since the first diagnosis of cancer, and here is what I found.

- *Chemotherapies—5 different drugs—60 total doses*
- *Radiation—28 exposures*
- *CT scans—51*
- *PET scans—2*
- *One of the chemotherapies I have had is known to cause MDS—I have it.*[49]
- *One of the chemotherapies I have had is known to cause hearing loss—I wear hearing aids (but in all fairness I used to listen to loud rock and roll, and we did not use earplugs in the Army at the firing range).*
- *CT scans are known to cause cancer—is the node in my left lung an awakened cancer from my past, or is it a result of so many CT scans? We will never know.*

These are the reasons we have chosen alternative medicine.

(At the time we were oblivious to the cumulative effects of all that radiation from the scans.)

Journal entry by DIANE HUSSEY—6/17/2011

Today is the first day of the rest of our lives. Yep, that saying is back. But it is true. Today Jerry started the Budwig diet—we both did. It doesn't sound all that appetizing, but it actually tasted quite good! Like children we fought over who got to lick the spoon and spatula! We had it for lunch as well as dinner. He should have it twice a day, and I will have it once a day to support him. It is a lifestyle change.

He's been doing a lot of reading about the Budwig diet, what's good for us and what is not. He informed me that our nonstick cookware is not good for us, so we went out and bought stainless so I can cook, and he can eat. :) He is embracing natural health 100 percent!

Tomorrow we join the organic food co-op and put in our order.

We are having more fun than you could believe. I felt a whole lot of uncertainty about the stem cell transplant and Jerry being in a hospital four to six weeks. The hospital is about sixty-five miles away. . . . Now we can just

---

[49] We now know that three chemotherapies Jerry had may contribute to or cause MDS.

focus on Jerry getting well.

So, we are rearranging our lives, and coming together to fight this battle together, and two ARE stronger than one.

As you go through this journey called life, take time to smell the roses and enjoy it!

LIVE, LAUGH, LOVE!

We Have a Plan!—Journal entry by DIANE HUSSEY—6/21/2011

We always seem to find the humor in the journey, and we are laughing at the title of today's post. Since the bone marrow transplant was cancelled, we had to return to the BMTC to pick up the PET scan and other paperwork. Interestingly enough, we ran into the surgeon, Dr. Port, in the hall. He asked, "What's happening?" We told him the bone marrow transplant was off, and why. He seemed sad as he told us, "But I had a plan!"

I told him no offense, but I believed God has a better plan for us.

So, what's the plan?

We're heading to Spain for twenty days at the Budwig Center. We believe they have the best alternative treatment plan for Jerry, and we are believing it was part of God's plan all along.

We are firming up the date and will let you know the details. Always remember, as you travel this road we call life, enjoy the journey!

Chapter 12

Autumn 2017—The Quest for Truth:

Cancer Four, Continued, and Cancer Five

From the five-inch stack of files, I pulled out the medical records related to the bone marrow transplant. With a warm cup of tea on the kitchen table before me, I paused and took a deep breath. *Why do I continue to put myself through this?* It had been difficult enough to read and relive the emotional journey documented in Jerry's CaringBridge journal.

I closed my eyes, hoping and praying I wouldn't find anything else. But then again, I'd never expected to find what I'd found with the previous investigations.

I downed some tea and dug in.

March 22, 2011, had been our initial appointment with the bone marrow transplant doctor, Dr. BMT. As I scanned his notes, I came across information that I really don't believe Jerry and I had heard before. There was a lot to process. Had Dr. BMT really told us this?

HUSSEY JERRY   MC#:
Diagnosis: sMDS   Primary BMT MD:

Triage Assessment

Assessment Date: 03/22/2011	Reason: Triage	Assessor:	RN, BSN
Height (In): 71.00		MD:	MD
Weight (kg): 101.75			
BP: 135/65			
Temperature: 97.70			
Pulse: 101			

Examination:
see progress note of same date

Laboratory Tests: 3/22/11: WBC 2.21, Hgb 11.3, plt 51
Performance Status: 90

Assessment:
his is a 62 years old male with MDS - RAEB -1 High risk disease based on WHO classification. His WHO Prognostic Scoring System (WPSS) Score was 5. Risk of AML progression and early mortality is very high. The median survival for this risk group is 12 months with cumulative probability of transformation to AML at 2-yr and 5-yr of 79% and 100% respectively. Of note, he also has therapy related MDS which also worsens his prognosis.
I have a long discussion with the patient regarding the treatment options which included but not limited to clinical trials, hypomethylating agents, AML-type chemotherapy, best supportive care and allogeneic Stem Cell Transplantation. With a goal of achieving long term survival, allogeneic stem cell transplant would be the preferred treatment option with the understanding that this could associated with significant morbidity and mortality from the treatment. I also discussed with the patient the nature of his disease, the prognosis and the rationale of allogeneic stem cell transplant as well as acute and chronic complications include but not limited to acute and chronic graft versus host disease.

Plans:
After the consultation, we were advised by the patient to proceed with obtaining HLA typing for the patient and his only sibling. Unfortunately, his sibling was not a match and we have obtained informed consent from the patient to proceed with a formal unrelated donor search. The preliminary search is very encouraging though it may take a few weeks to identify a suitable donor. It will be reasonable to consider treating him with a hypomethylating agent before we can take him to transplant. I will discuss with patient and Dr.

Signed _____   Signed _____

Date: _____ Time _____   Date: _____ Time: _____

from March 22, 2011, document

". . . Risk of AML (acute myeloid leukemia) progression and early mortality is very high. The median survival for this risk group is 12 months with cumulative probability of transformation to AML at 2-yr and 5-yr of 79 percent and 100 percent respectively. Of note, he also has therapy related MDS which also worsens his prognosis."

It felt like a short circuit in my brain. *Risk of leukemia progression . . . Early mortality very high . . . Median survival **twelve** months.* Had the doctor really told us this? I reflected on the office visit, only remembering that we had been told a bone barrow transplant was our best hope.

Needing to know a little more about AML, I accessed the Internet.

Acute myeloid leukemia. *Acute* means that this leukemia can progress quickly if not treated and would probably be fatal in a few months. *Myeloid* refers to the type of cell this leukemia starts from.

Apparently, most cases of AML develop from cells that would turn into white blood cells (other than lymphocytes).[50]

I don't remember *any* mention of Jerry being at high risk for AML or leukemia. All I remember is the doctor talking about MDS which, in my mind (and I believe in Jerry's as well), was conquerable. I'm sure if the doctor had said *leukemia*, we'd have both reacted differently—far more fearful and concerned.

I continued to read the report.

"I have (sic) a long discussion with the patient regarding the treatment options which included but not limited to clinical trials, hypomethylating agents, AML-type chemotherapy, best supportive care and allogeneic Stem Cell Transplantation."

Time out—that's not true. We were at a facility that specialized in bone marrow/stem cell transplants, specifically for that possibility alone. There was no discussion of clinical trials, chemotherapy, or other potential types of care.

Continuing with the report: "With a goal of achieving long term survival, allogeneic stem cell transplant would be the preferred treatment option with the understanding that this could [be] associated with significant morbidity and mortality from the treatment."

Again, the stem cell transplant itself could cause "significant morbidity and mortality"? It's the second time it appears in the report, but that was never verbalized to Jerry and me. During the appointment, we were sold on the hype

---

[50] https://www.cancer.org/cancer/acute-myeloid-leukemia/about/what-is-aml.html

and hope of the bone marrow transplant—Dr. BMT represented it optimistically and positively. Jerry felt it was his only option, and a good option.

I forced myself to keep reading.

"I also discussed with the patient the nature of his disease, the prognosis and rationale of allogeneic stem cell transplant as well as acute and chronic complications include[ing] but not limited to acute and chronic graft versus host disease."

Prognosis of the transplant? Graft versus host disease? I studied the report again. *If* the doctor had given us the facts as he had written them, would we have been so eager to move forward? We'd understood that Jerry might be in the hospital for six weeks, then going to the BMTC for tests twice a week for quite some time. But all of that to perhaps get twelve months?

We weren't willing to settle for "maybe two and a half years" with the experimental treatment. Why would we settle for twelve months?

It boggled my mind to read all that doctor BMT had listed in his report.

As I've reviewed Jerry's medical records, I've found that oncologists tend not to volunteer certain information to patients, but they certainly try to cover themselves in their medical reports from all potential litigation.

I examined the copies of all the BMT paperwork we'd been given that Jerry had signed: Financial Responsibility Agreement, Authorization to Discuss Medical Information, HIPPA, Patient Demographics, Transplant Program Treatment Synopsis, Policies and Procedures, Definitions, Materials, Personnel, Procedure, and Calculations. Nowhere, in any of our copies, does the information reflect what Dr. BMT wrote in his Assessment in Jerry's medical record.

What, if anything, was I going to find next? My thoughts kept wandering back to the report. I just couldn't shake the feeling that we'd been sold a bill of goods.

Flipping through the pages of labs, test results, appointments, and schedules began to frazzle my brain. I was "sifting," but what was I looking for?

And then I saw it—the word *spiculations*, on the 6/2/2011 CT scan. I remembered from Jerry's first lung cancer that spiculated had meant a tissue lump with spikes on the surface. What had that indicated? I looked it up again.

> A spiculated edge is an independent predictor of malignancy in a lung nodule.[51]

---

[51] http://www.clevelandclinicmeded.com/medicalpubs/diseasemanagement/hematology-oncology/pulmonary-nodules/

This CT scan, which had been done shortly after the bone marrow donor had been found, the day Jerry was rushed to the emergency department with a-fib, showed a "1.2 x 0.9 cm, round soft tissue density nodule seen in the anterior left upper lobe with subtle *spiculations*."

Fussey, Jerry (MR #   )

considered enlarged by CT criteria.

Postsurgical changes are seen from prior right upper lobectomy with surgical clips along the upper posterior right mediastinum, atelectasis and mild fibrotic changes. A 1.2 x 0.9 cm, round soft tissue density nodule seen in the anterior left upper lobe with subtle spiculations (image 70/4). No other definite nodules are identified. There is mild

from June 2, 2011, document (page 2)

But wait, that meant that as early as June 2, 2011, Dr. BMT had to have known that the BMT would probably be cancelled!

A few paragraphs down the page, the truth stared at me. "Left upper lobe nodule. Correlation with prior imaging is recommended to assess if this is a new finding. *Underlying malignancy cannot be excluded*, especially in this patient with history of lung cancer. . . . Follow-up is recommended."

IMPRESSION:

1. Negative for pulmonary embolism. These results were verbally reported by   , M.D. to   , M.D. at 1715 hrs on 6/2/11.

2. Left upper lobe nodule. Correlation with prior imaging is recommended to assess if this is a new finding. Underlying malignancy cannot be excluded, especially in this patient with history of lung cancer.

3. Post surgical changes from prior right upper lobectomy.

4. Borderline prominent right subcarinal lymph node. Follow-up is recommended.

from June 2, 2011, document (page 2)

The next CT scan, taken five days afterward, stopped me in my tracks.

In the left lung, there is a dominant pulmonary nodule at the anterior medial aspect of the left upper lobe on image 42/4. This nodule measures 1.3 x 1.1 cm, previously measuring 0.8 x 0.8 cm and appearing less solid. No other left-sided pulmonary nodules are identified. There is no

from June 7, 2011, document (page 2)

"In the left lung . . . This nodule measures 1.3 x 1.1 cm, previously measuring 0.8 x 0.8 cm. . . ."

Wait. What? The CT from five days prior had measured the nodule at 1.2 x 0.9 cm. What previous measurement of "0.8 x 0.8 cm" was this referring to? Just how long had they known about this nodule?

I can't begin to count the days, hours, and attempts to find the CT scan documenting the 0.8 x 0.8 cm left lung nodule. Had it been done under Dr. PM or at the BMTC?

More than a year passed. During the last edit, I finally found it. I couldn't believe how I'd missed it, though I'd been looking for a 0.8 x 0.8 cm nodule in the left lobe. And there it was, in the June 2, 2011, CT scan, mentioned in relation to the right lobe.

regions. However, there is a right subcarinal lymph node which measures approximately 8 mm in short access (series 4 image 62). This is not

Hussey, Jerry (MR #   ) Printed by   , RN [   ] at 6/6/11 9:54 ... Page 1 of

from June 2, 2011, document (page 1)

Hussey, Jerry (MR #   )

considered enlarged by CT criteria.

Postsurgical changes are seen from prior right upper lobectomy with surgical clips along the upper posterior right mediastinum, atelectasis and mild fibrotic changes. A 1.2 x 0.9 cm, round soft tissue density nodule seen in the anterior left upper lobe with subtle spiculations (image 70/4). No other definite nodules are identified. There is mild

from June 2, 2011, document (page 2)

"...*Right* subcarinal lymph node which measures approximately 8 mm..." Yes, 8 mm is the same as 0.8 x 0.8 cm, so I felt foolish not figuring that out sooner, but how incompetent was the author of the June 7, 2011, report?

So, the report compared a *pulmonary nodule on the left* side to a *subcarinal lymph node from the right side*. Unbelievable! And doctors and others rely on these records?

When I turned to page 3 of the June 7, 2011, document, even that issue faded to the background.

IMPRESSION:
1. Interval increase in size of left upper lobe pulmonary nodule when compared to the outside CT from a year ago. This nodule also appears to be more solid on the current CT. This is suspicious for neoplasm. This could be further evaluated with percutaneous biopsy or PET scan.

from June 7, 2011, document (page 3)

". . . Increase in size of left upper lobe pulmonary nodule when compared to the outside CT from *a year ago*."

That would have been under Dr. PM's watch. Why hadn't he mentioned it? (Again, an issue with a nodule in the lung that wasn't shared with us until much later. Clearly there's a pattern here!)

So, Dr. PM had known about this lung nodule for eight months and chosen not to follow up with a CT scan?

I retrieved the stack of records from Dr. PM. Because I often worked in my kitchen, all of Jerry's records had become a permanent decoration on the counter, stacked according to the cancer and then the doctor/hospital.

How had I missed reading about the new lung nodule in these records? Because the paperwork is totally mind-numbing? Where was the scan Jerry should have had in January or February? There wasn't one. Why? Delving deeper into the records from the previous year, I found that Dr. PM had recommended Jerry graduate from CT scans every six months to annually.

But wouldn't it make sense that finding a new nodule on 7/9/2010 should override that decision?

Accession #: CT-	Procedure Name: CT Chest W/O Contrast		Exam Date 7/9/10 9:27:40	Ordering Physician:

Results
HISTORY: Lung cancer

COMPARISON: 01/29/2010

TECHNIQUE: Helically acquired axial images were obtained through the chest without IV contrast as per request per the ordering physician. Additional sagittal and coronal reformatted images of the chest were performed.

FINDINGS: No definite axillary, mediastinal or hilar lymphadenopathy is identified. Postoperative changes are again identified within the right upper hemithorax, with associated post radiation change as well. Probable scarring is present in the right lower hemithorax. A 3 mm nodule is present the medial aspect of the left upper lobe. No new suspicious parenchymal nodular densities or focal infiltrates are identified.

Evaluation of the unenhanced upper abdomen demonstrates decreased attenuation of the liver, suggestive of fatty infiltration.

Copies to:

Print Date: 06/06/11
Print Time: 4:02 PM   Page 1 of 2

from July 9, 2010, document

Settle down, Diane. The new nodule had been only 3 mm, which is very tiny, not even the size of a bb. Neither the radiologist nor Dr. PM had seen characteristics at that time to indicate this nodule might become cancerous. It's possible I was overreacting.

Though again, with Jerry's history, wouldn't it make sense that finding this nodule would prompt the oncologist to keep an eye on it more often than once a year?

Also, this July 9, 2010, report meant that Dr. BMT, who'd obtained all of Jerry's records from Dr. PM, had to have known about this new lung nodule from the beginning (which had been confirmed in the BMTC intake history, a history so detailed that it had gone all the way back to Jerry's original cancer and oncologist in San Antonio).

Why hadn't Dr. BMT ordered a CT scan prior to accepting Jerry to the BMT program in late March 2011? He'd known that Dr. PM had found this lung nodule the year prior and that Jerry had a history of two previous lung cancers. The questions spun inside my head as I confirmed it with the first CT scan done at the BMTC on 6/2/2011.

There it was, in writing, under Comparison.

Narrative:
CT CHEST WITH CONTRAST-PE PROTOCOL.

DATE: 06/02/11 16:46:00.

INDICATION: 61-year-old male with new onset nature fibrillation with elevated d-dimer. Per the electronic medical record, the patient has a history of myelodysplastic syndrome and lung cancer status post lobectomy.

COMPARISON: No comparisons are available at this institution.

---

from June 2, 2011, document (page 1)

"No comparisons (CT scans) are available at this institution." In other words, *We haven't done a CT scan on this patient.* That note had been made just eleven days before the BMT was cancelled.

I skimmed back through Jerry's CaringBridge posts. On May 19, 2011, he'd written, *"Between now and June 15, I will have four trips to the bone marrow transplant center for tests and checkups. I will get the alphabet soup of tests: EEG, EKG, CT, and whatever else they think of."* But on May 25, 2011, he'd journaled, *"Actually, the tests went well, and I'm glad to know my heart is healthy and beating the way it is supposed to beat. I had an EKG, and all of my valves and other functions are completely normal."* Jerry hadn't mentioned getting a CT scan. Even at that point, May 25, 2011, just three weeks before

June 15 when Jerry was to start the bone marrow transplant process, the BMTC still hadn't ordered any CT scan.

My ire mounted. I found it particularly disturbing that the BMTC did not order a CT scan prior to accepting Jerry into the BMT program, particularly since the most recent CT scan had been almost a year before. We'd been told several times that the BMTC would not accept patients who they believed had a poor (hopeless) prognosis.

Once that cognition clicked into my mental chamber, the thoughts machine-gunned:

- Before Jerry had been accepted to the BMT program, Dr. BMT had obtained Jerry's records from Dr. PM, including all CT scans.
- The most recent CT scan, from nearly a year ago, revealed the lung nodule.
- Dr. BMT had known about the lung nodule from day one.
- The "subtle spiculations" on the nodule, noted on June 2, 2011, appeared to be a recent development.
- As of the June 2, 2011, CT scan, Dr. BMT had known Jerry's lung nodule was likely cancerous.
- The June 7, 2011, page 3, CT scan read, "This could be further evaluated with percutaneous biopsy or PET scan."
- On June 9, 2011, during our appointment with Dr. BMT and the transplant team, the doctor had shared the news. "Jerry, the CT scan showed a suspicious spot in the upper left lobe of your lung that has started to grow. We will need to do a PET scan to assess whether it is cancer, which would terminate the transplant."

So, <u>the BMT team had been fully aware of the nodule from the get-go in late March,</u> but *they hadn't even checked for cancer* <u>until June 2011</u>.

My anger continued to rise. If they didn't accept patients with poor prognosis, then why, with Jerry's history, hadn't Dr. BMT ordered a CT scan on the nodule *before* they'd accepted Jerry into the program? A 3 mm nodule could easily be a larger and cancerous nodule within a year.

For two and a half months, Jerry had gone through every test imaginable, including an excruciating bone marrow biopsy, and so had his would-be donor. Jerry had gone through every test, except a CT scan on his lung.

Why?

As detailed as Dr. BMT had been, even down to the precise statistics he'd specified in Jerry's records, and as detailed as every step of the BMT process had been, I couldn't believe the lack of an updated CT scan had been an oversight, a case of a patient's testing falling through the cracks. It was virtually impossible that it had been negligence.

My thoughts turned sarcastic. *Had there been a medical reason why Dr. BMT had determined, without testing, that the new lung nodule from a year ago couldn't possibly have become cancerous?*

I frowned at the stack of insurance paperwork, knowing that if the BMTC had done that *one* test two and a half months earlier, tens of thousands of dollars that had been paid by our insurance company could have been saved.

The June 2, 2011, CT scan had found indications of cancer. Eleven days had passed before the PET scan had been done on June 13, 2011, . . . coincidentally after Dr. BMT had made sure Jerry had fulfilled all the appointments they'd planned and could bill.

Call me cynical, *or* consider that we received a fax confirming the nodule was consistent with malignancy later the same day of the PET scan. That fax had been the last communication we received from the BMTC. Because there had been nothing else they could do, or bill for, Jerry had been dropped like a hot potato.

The thought assaulted my brain: That was it. The hospital and its doctors had reaped a substantial profit with all the doctor appointments, tests, labs, and everything else they'd billed for.

Since the bone marrow transplant had been cancelled instantly once the nodule had proved cancerous, just two days prior to the target date for Jerry to be admitted to the hospital, clearly none of the BMT process would have taken place had the nodule been found to be cancerous at the beginning.

How could the reason be anything but financial gain?

In my mind, no doubt, we'd been sold a bill of goods.

☐

It was almost more than I could bear. Everything had to be set aside for a while so I could regroup and tackle it again. Thankfully, when I jumped back in, I found a document that made me smile—the results of Jerry's pre-bone marrow transplant psych test. It delighted me so much that I read it a couple of times.

"Impressions and Recommendations: Mr. Hussey is experiencing an appropriate level of health-related concern but does not appear to be experiencing psychological distress at this time. He has a history of coping well with major life stressors and multiple cancer diagnoses, and appears to be coping very well at present. He has good social support which he utilizes appropriately."

That's my Jerry.

Not to brag, but here it is, in the document.

> **Impressions and Recommendations:** Mr. Hussey is experiencing an appropriate level of health-related concern but does not appear to be experiencing psychological distress at this time. He has a history of coping well with major life stressors and multiple cancer diagnoses, and appears to be coping very well at present. He has good social support which he utilizes appropriately. Mr. Hussey

from June 2, 2011, document (page 3)

It's kind of funny how reading Jerry's psychological report reminded me how normal and wonderful he truly was. Such a good guy! Love was in the air! □

Around this same time, I found a copy of our wedding ceremony tucked among photographs. When we married in 1972, it wasn't uncommon for couples to write their own wedding ceremonies. At the time, I had selected portions of at least three ceremonies and had woven them together. Jerry had been in the Army Reserves and off serving his two-week summer camp obligation while I worked away on our service. It still makes my heart happy as I read it and reflect on our marriage.

Here the bonds of marriage are formed. For marriage, which is always spoken of as a bond, becomes actually, in this stage, many bonds, many strands of different texture and strength, making up a web that is taut and firm.

The web is fashioned of love. Yes, but many kinds of love: romantic love at first, then a slow growing devotion, and playing through these, a constantly rippling companionship. It is made of loyalties, and interdependencies, and shared experiences. It is woven of memories of meetings and conflicts, of triumphs and disappointments.

It is a web of communication, a common language, and the acceptance of lack of language too. A knowledge of likes and dislikes, of habits and reactions, both physical and mental. It is a web of instincts and institutions and known exchanges.

> The web of marriage is made by closeness, in the day-to-day
> living side by side, looking outward and working outward in the
> same direction. It is woven in space and in time of the substance
> of life itself.

Yes, every sentence resonated with me and stirred a warmth within. I reread and savored the words, visualizing the weaving of the bonds to create a web, taut and firm. A web of love and of all the components of life. We truly were blessed, and I realized we had fulfilled the prophecy we'd had the minister speak over our marriage.

Much of that blessing came from our attitudes and decisions. We didn't fight, and we thought before we spoke. Life wasn't always easy, but we made the choice to weather the storms together. As I pondered the words once more before moving on, I realized how God had prepared us as a team early on for what would be the biggest challenge of our lives.

□

All of the chemotherapy, radiation, and surgery had been very hard on Jerry. My preferences had been for natural health. Although I will take a moment and attempt to present the contrast between the two approaches honestly, I again confess my bias.

Conventional doctors are trained to treat symptoms with medicine or surgery, and there are times their medical intervention is necessary and lifesaving. However, medical doctors receive almost no education in nutrition or disease prevention.

General practitioners often refer patients to specialists because of the complexity of issues involving different areas of the body. Since specialists, well, specialize, we often must see more than one for our issues. Because each only treats one area of the body—heart, digestion, kidneys, bones, or you name the body part—doctors usually cannot, or will not, address issues that fall outside their area of expertise. When a patient has two or more doctors, for example a kidney doctor (nephrologist) and oncologist, they may conflict on their recommended treatments.

Often we hear that doctors don't know what is wrong with someone. Symptoms may arise that befuddle a specialist because the cause is not in his area of expertise, and they order test after test to try to diagnose the problem.

Could it be that they are so specialized that when they focus on one portion of the body, that they don't understand how the body works as a whole?

We do need them, though. The medical community has incredible technology and resources that can help us when we've had an accident, many illnesses and diseases, or emergency situations. Doctors are also helpful when we have ignored and allowed our health to deteriorate to a level that is dangerous, such as heart disease. I know many people who wouldn't be alive without doctors, surgeons, nurses, paramedics, therapists, and a host of other medical professionals and technologies.

I have many concerns, however, with our medical system, but rather than start down that road, I will politely say that medicine, technology, and treatment should be applied wisely and with discernment, instead of indiscriminately or routinely amid a collective refusal to gain knowledge of natural, non-pharmaceutical options.

Not to lay blame entirely on the medical community. We, as consumers, also bear responsibility. There are many who run to the doctor over every illness and think they need medication because the pharmaceutical commercials encourage us to ask our doctors for pills to take care of a multitude of issues. Pay no attention to the side effects that are quickly mentioned, which are often worse than the malady they are designed to help.

Often when a doctor issues a prescription, we take it without questioning the doctor or pharmacist. Instead, we should be actively engaged in our health, inquiring about the side effects and long-term ramifications of the drug, tests, or treatments. We should request full disclosure of potential consequences of all recommended treatment options.

In contrast, naturopaths, or alternative health practitioners, seek to find and address the *root cause* of an illness or affliction. They focus on the whole person—all areas of the body, plus the mind and spirit. The goal is to strengthen the immune system through detoxing, diet, and many other methods. Our bodies have the amazing ability to heal themselves if we give them what they need and stop abusing them.

Natural health works to harness our body's own healing ability, using a wide variety of therapies: nutrition, herbs, water, air, essential oils, massage, acupuncture, and electro-medicine, to name a few. Many involved with holistic or integrative health understand how the whole body works together, even to the cellular level. Attention to exercise and mental/emotional health can also help us keep our bodies and immune systems healthy, making us less susceptible to disease.

There are many other therapies, too numerous to mention, and options currently available that may not have been available in 2011. I have friends who swear about the effectiveness of CBD oil and/or medical marijuana (among others) for cancer and other health issues. Rather than trying to address new alternatives, I am limiting discussion to what we knew, and methods recommended that we employed.

Both conventional and holistic approaches are clinically proven and have their merits. Natural health is more proactive and tends to treat from the inside out, whereas conventional medicine tends to be reactive and treat from the outside in, such as administering pharmaceutical drugs.

To simply differentiate between health care practitioners: conventional doctors chase and treat symptoms. Holistic or alternative health care practitioners seek the origins of the issue and address the cause. A natural approach makes so much more sense.

And giving your body what it needs to heal, while avoiding substances and situations that contribute to illness, makes the most sense of all.

Chapter 13
Cancer Simplified—The Science

One of my goals all along has been to help take the mystery out of cancer in order to empower you, the reader. My sifting through vast amounts of information has yielded nuggets that I will attempt to share in understandable concepts. That makes this one of the most important chapters in the book.

Four Basic Causes of Cancer

Let's start out simply, based on Jerry and my research and the *Budwig Center Wellness Cancer Guide*[52] we received in 2011.

We came to understand that there are four causes of cancer, and that the causes are interconnected. While all four of these conditions contribute to cancer growing and spreading, it's vital to gain understanding at the cellular level. The following is *extremely* simplified.

- **Weakened Immune System:** We are only as healthy as the majority of our cells. Healthy cells equal a healthy immune system and ultimately a healthy body. Cells need good food, water, and oxygen to be healthy individually, and collectively.

    A strong immune system consistently targets and kills individual cancer cells.

- **Toxins:** When we have too much of something, it's considered toxic or poisonous. We are constantly exposed to toxins/poisons through chemicals, pesticides, herbicides, plastics, polluted air, polluted water, electronic pollution, and GMOs (genetically modified organisms— unnatural, lab-generated alterations to the plants and animals we eat).

    Basically, there are four ways we get poisoned: by what we ingest, inhale, absorb through our skin, and what we inject or is injected into us.

    Here are just a few things that can harm us due to exposure or accumulative exposure:

---

[52] http://www.budwigcenter.com

- ▫ <u>ingested</u>: chlorine and other chemicals in our water (I'll address this shortly.)
- ▫ <u>inhaled</u>: off-gassing from plastics (especially from cars baking in the sun—open doors and/or roll down windows to air out)
- ▫ <u>absorbed through the skin</u>: the chemicals in many detergents, fabric softeners, soaps, shampoos, lotions, and makeup (be sure to read labels and research ingredients, then find nontoxic alternative products)
- ▫ <u>injected</u>: vaccinations (Vaccinations are controversial but are included for your consideration and personal research. Some have been, largely, beneficial. Others have resulted in an unacceptable amount of personal harm.)

Many people may hear "injected" and think of a drug addict shooting illegal drugs into their veins and obviously how harmful that can be. But keep in mind that chemotherapy is injected poison designed to kill cells.

Toxins impact the health and viability of cells, and sick cells weaken our immune system. That leads to sick organs and systems, diseases, or general ill health.

Thankfully, our body can remove toxins if we drink enough healthy water, exercise, and make a concerted effort, sometimes healing one organ at a time.

- **Improper Diet:** When we don't eat as we should, it creates a nutrient deficiency. If our cells don't receive enough of what they need to function properly, the cells, organs, and entire body can become sick or diseased. Today we are generally deficient in vitamins, minerals, and other nutrients, which we should get through food or supplementation. Even a deficiency in just one nutrient, such as iodine, can affect our health.

Continuing to focus on iodine as an example, did you know that iodine consumption has plummeted 50 percent since 1970 and has corresponded with a dramatic increase in breast and prostate cancers?

The immune system needs need iodine to facilitate cell death in breast cancer and to suppress tumor growth.

Studies show that iodine deficiency is a worldwide epidemic, often affecting women of reproductive age. This could not only increase their risk of cancer but also could cause complications during pregnancy and in fetal development.

Additionally, deficiency of iodine has been found to influence the occurrence of other cancers. For instance, in the country Turkey, gastric cancers are most common in areas where iodine deficiency is high.

However, increased iodine intake over the past several years has been strongly correlated with a reduction in stomach cancers. Researchers have attributed the low rate of breast cancer in Japan to high dietary iodine (and selenium).[53]

Eating unhealthy foods—improper diet—also adds to the toxins in our bodies, weakening our immune system.

- **Oxygen Deprivation:** In 1931, Dr. Otto Warburg received his Nobel Prize for proving that an underlying cause of cancer is low levels of oxygen in the cells. In the article "The Prime Cause and Prevention of Cancer," he stated, "The cause of cancer is no longer a mystery. We know it occurs whenever any cell is denied 60 percent of its oxygen requirements."[54]

So how does that happen? The simplified explanation is that normal cells use oxygen efficiently to create energy. If cancer cells don't have sufficient oxygen, they resort to fermentation, which is very inefficient and creates tremendous amounts of waste.

Or, simply put, cancer cells are sick, low-oxygen cells that are not functioning properly.

---

[53] https://thetruthaboutcancer.com/low-iodine-cancer/
[54] https://www.cancerfightingstrategies.com/oxygen-and-cancer.html

Toxins and improper diet contribute to oxygen deprivation in the cells, weakening the immune system so it can't kill cancer. It's a vicious cycle.

A couple of other areas worth mentioning, which we can control simply enough, impact our health both on the cellular and systemic (system-wide) levels.

Dehydration: We need plenty of healthy water every day to deliver oxygen and nutrients to all the cells in our body. Coffee, tea, soda, energy drinks, and alcohol do *not* hydrate the cells and can make them sick due to the sugar, sugar substitutes, and other substances.

Lymph system: Basically our lymph system is the garbage-collection system in our body. Unlike our circulatory system, which has a heart to pump the blood, our lymph system functions by our body movement. That means exercise is critical. Lymph fluid is approximately 95 percent water, so we need to stay well hydrated to allow this line of defense in our body to function optimally.

Which symptoms might signify a congested lymph system? Stiffness, especially in the morning, fatigue, itchy and dry skin, bloating, brain fog, swollen glands, stubborn weight gain, chronic sinusitis, sore throats, colds, or ear issues, to name a few.

During our cancer four brouhaha, Jerry finally realized just how critical health and nutrition are when battling cancer, and I learned more about how nutrition specifically relates to the disease. As a result we both made lifestyle changes and much healthier choices.

I'll share strategies for addressing cancer shortly. But first I'll give a little more information regarding factors that contribute to cancer and related considerations that are essential to understand.

Genetics and Cancer

As we move further into understanding cancer, it's important to pause and get the facts on genetics. Many people believe they are predisposed to get cancer because it "runs in the family." Statistically, that doesn't line up. From the National Cancer Institute, inherited mutations causing cancer only "play a role in about 5 to 10 percent of all cancers."[55]

Then why does it seem to run in families? Because we are far more impacted by family-of-origin tendencies, including where we live, what we eat,

---

[55] https://www.cancer.gov/about-cancer/causes-prevention/genetics

drink, the air we breathe, smoking, stress, work, how much we exercise, and other environmental and societal factors, than by cancer "genetics."

Stop for a moment and consider your birth family. If they smoked, you were subjected to second-hand smoke, and you were more likely to smoke too. Where was your home? In the city near heavily traveled roadways with prolonged rush hours and polluted air? Or rural where agricultural chemicals filled the soil and air? Near high-voltage power lines? Were your family dynamics filled with strife and stress? Did you eat more healthy, nutritious food or junk food? Factoring in all those elements, doesn't it make sense that sharing the same environment would impact our health to make it appear as if cancer runs in the family?

(I'm not dismissing that some breast, ovarian, colorectal, and prostate cancers are reported to be hereditary, but these gene-influenced cancers represent just a small percentage of all types and incidences of cancer. My recommendation for anyone who has one of these cancers is to actively engage in practices that promote health and wellness, which include strengthening your immune system and remaining ever vigilant regarding your health.)

Our jobs can also impact our odds of getting cancer. Certain industries have more chemical, radiation, or electronics exposure. Malignant mesothelioma is a classic example of cancer related to work or environment. Will you find your job listed in the article "15 Jobs That Put You at a Higher Risk for Cancer?"[56] Some may seem obvious, like manufacturing rubber, plastics, or a chemical factory worker. But working in the trades (construction, mechanic, and metalworking) are also listed. The chemicals used in personal care by hairdressers, barbers, and nail technicians are hazardous and put those professions on the list. Even pilots and those involved in high-stress jobs make it into the top fifteen.

There is no magic answer as to why some get cancer and others don't, but we have far more ability to impact our odds of getting or not getting cancer than we have been led to believe. As cardiologist Donald Lloyd-Jones states, "For most people, a healthy lifestyle trumps inherited risk."[57]

Ultimately, the risk of cancer comes down to choices and personal responsibility. Since that is the case, we have the power to take control of our health and not live in fear. Some will be thankful and embrace the opportunity to have more control over their life, making changes with an attitude that fosters

---

[56] https://www.cheatsheet.com/money-career/jobs-put-higher-cancer-risk.html/
[57] https://www.webmd.com/healthy-aging/features/genes-or-lifestyle

healthy living. Others will continue to make unhealthy choices and wonder why they're sick.

This May Be the One, Root Cause of Cancer

It seems as if everyone is concerned about cancer, but most people feel helpless and clueless. The medical community likes to keep it a huge mystery.

As I was researching the causes of cancer in 2017, I became fascinated while studying the article "What Causes Cancer?"[58] from CancerTutor.com. I hope this brief overview gives you the desire to search beyond what I present here.

Previously I provided four general causes of cancer: a weakened immune system, toxins, improper diet, and oxygen deprivation. Cancer Tutor offers what I believe to be the most comprehensive, root explanation of the causes.

The following is highly edited to provide a *concept*, with extremely simplified explanations to ensure easiest understanding. Again, I encourage you to visit this invaluable website.

Cancer Tutor proposes that microbes and parasites are the culprits that initiate cancer by invading the cells, organs, or the bloodstream. To understand cancer, it is essential to differentiate between cancer at the cellular and systemic levels.

First, let's look at cancer at the *cellular* level and how microbes create cancer. (I repeat, this is ultra-simplified!)

All cells need food—glucose. In a normal, healthy cell, some of the glucose is used by the cell to make energy (ATP—adenosine triphosphate). In the process, oxygen is consumed, and carbon dioxide and water are formed (easily eliminated by the body). Energy production is very high.

Cancer cells, by comparison (and by definition), are low ATP energy cells. Although cancer cells consume as much as 15 times more glucose than a normal cell, they produce only 5 percent of the energy. Thus, they create a tremendous amount of waste. Our bodies have an ability to handle it, to a point.

If we look ahead in time to understand the whole cycle when the body is extremely compromised and the cancer is in an advanced state, we will begin to understand how the devastation of cancer decimates the body with an avalanche of waste.

The cellular waste travels through the bloodstream to the liver where it is converted into glucose, which is transported back to the cells.

---

[58] https://www.cancertutor.com/what_causes_cancer/

The cycle starts again, and it is this "ping pong ball" cycle (called the lactic acid cycle or cachexia cycle) that ramps up when cancer is in an advanced state. It causes weight loss and is what kills about half of all cancer patients because so much energy is consumed at both ends of the cycle. (Cachexia is the weight loss and wasting of muscle tissue due to severe chronic illness. This cycle can be broken, although the medical community offers no answers for this vicious cycle. Again, CancerTutor.com is a good resource.)

If that isn't bad enough, the lactic acid also blocks many key nutrients from getting to the cancer cells in the first place. And finally, cancer microbes, which I'll discuss in a moment, also excrete enzymes that coat the outside of the cancer cells. This coating of enzymes blocks the immune system from identifying the cancer cells as being cancerous.

One of my friends says it best: Cancer is just evil.

So, how do microbes get into a cell? Briefly, it is theorized that H. pylori bacteria can drill into a cell wall to escape overly acidic blood. Also, asbestos and the chemicals in tobacco can cut a cell's membrane. Once a cell's membrane is compromised, microbes can move in. Once inside a cell, they intercept the glucose that the cell needs. The microbes excrete mycotoxins (waste), which are highly acidic.

Thus, the cells that contain microbes don't get the food they need, plus they now live in a sea of filth (i.e., mycotoxins), so the cells become weak.

With that basic understanding, let's move on to cancer at the systemic level.

The pattern is very similar, with microbes and parasites getting inside of the cells of the organs. When inside an organ's cells, they intercept the glucose that the organ's cells need. The microbes excrete mycotoxins (waste), which are highly acidic.

The organ's cells don't get the food they need, plus they now live in a sea of filth (i.e., mycotoxins), so the organ becomes weak.

Then, because one or more major organs are weak, the immune system becomes weak.

When the immune system is weak, it cannot kill enough cancer cells, and the cancer cells grow out of control.

And finally, microbes that find safe dwelling in the organs will spread microbes to the bloodstream, and vice versa, thus potentially spreading cancer.

So, the incredibly simplified explanation: When cancer occurs at the cellular level, it creates a cycle to feed the cancer. When those cells are found in the organs, they can create a toxic environment that weakens the immune system.

The weakened immune system compromises our ability to fight against cancer, and the cycle continues.

How Cancerous Tumors Form and Metastasize

I often find it helpful to visualize, so let's use a simple analogy to show how a localized cancerous environment (mass, nodule, tumor) can form.

Imagine a race car on a hoist in a closed garage running full throttle, tires spinning and going nowhere. It's burning fuel and polluting the environment with its exhaust. If the garage is not tightly sealed, the exhaust can escape into the environment.

Like the race car, a cancer cell burns through glucose (fuel), creating a toxic environment, polluting the cell as well as the cells surrounding it.

Does it make sense that this can create a localized cancerous environment (tumor)? Plus, if the toxins are able to escape, they can wreak havoc by spreading cancer to other areas, or by feeding the cachexia cycle that consumes so much energy that the patient wastes away.

Now, cancer cells are also characterized by uncontrolled cell division. If the body's normal control mechanism (apoptosis) stops working (due to a weakened immune system), cancer cells don't die. Instead, they continue to grow rapidly, abnormally (mutate), and out of control.

These cancer cells become invasive and start to take over a part of the body (creating a tumor or mass) or spread to other areas (metastasize). The cancer cells have been given what they need to wage war on the body.

So, cancer happens at the cellular level, and a tumor or mass is cancer at the systemic level.

Apoptosis

A form of cell death in which a programmed sequence of events leads to the elimination of cells without releasing harmful substances into the surrounding area. Apoptosis plays a crucial role in developing and maintaining the health of the body by eliminating old cells, unnecessary cells, and unhealthy cells. The human body replaces perhaps one million cells per second. Too little or too much apoptosis can play a role in many diseases. When apoptosis does not work correctly, cells that should be eliminated may persist and become immortal, for example, in cancer and leukemia. When apoptosis works overly well, it kills too many cells and inflicts grave tissue damage. This is the case in strokes and neurodegenerative disorders such as Alzheimer's, Huntington's, and Parkinson's diseases.[59]

Blood cancer, on the other hand, is not a solid tumor, but occurs in the bone marrow and blood. These abnormal cells build up and crowd out normal cells, impacting the formation and development of white and red blood cells, hemoglobin, and platelets. The low level of normal blood cells can make it harder for the body to get oxygen to its tissues, control bleeding, and fight infection.

So, How Does One Best Fight, or Even Avoid, Cancer?

Here is the key concept (again ultra-simplified): *If we can build or maintain a healthy immune system so that it can deal with cancer at the **cellular** level, we can, in theory, fight off or avoid cancer at the **systemic** level.*

It isn't unheard of, however, for people who do all the "right" things to get cancer. Why? I can't answer that question, and it seems nobody can. But if we can help people understand enough about cancer that they can start to make the changes to keep them healthy, we have the potential to globally turn the tide on cancer.

Cancer and the Shady Side of the Internet

Before diving in to look deeper into natural health versus conventional medicine approaches to cancer, it's important to remember that the Internet is filled with an abundance of information, both accurate and inaccurate. When you research, then, discretion must be used. Often there appears to be a war between making information available for our benefit, and an attempt to suppress information with disinformation. When you research you'll find there is a lot of deception and misrepresentation from sources who have a lot to lose financially. It is vital that as you look, you consider the motivation. Ultimately, you will be the one to make the decision about what you believe.

Thankfully, a lot of information is now available on holistic, natural, functional, or integrative medicine (all are forms of alternative healing) on the Internet, and if that is what you are seeking, it is helpful to use one of those qualifying terms to try to differentiate it from conventional treatment.

---

[59] https://www.medicinenet.com/script/main/art.asp?articlekey=11287

For a very candid overview of the differences between the two main options, alternative and conventional, take the time to investigate Dr. Peter Glidden,[60] a doctor who is extremely outspoken regarding our medical system.

While you conduct your own research, I believe your confidence in our medical system will crack, like ours did.

As I've already shared, we learned a lot due to Jerry's cancer journey. I sought to understand medical terms and treatment, natural health, and anything else that seemed pertinent. It was extremely time-consuming and often emotionally charged. I became increasingly skeptical of conventional oncological medicine the more I explored and analyzed.

To ensure accuracy while writing the manuscript, I double- and triple-checked original sources used and quoted, often finding that there had been drastic changes. Some articles were no longer available. Others that reflected negatively on the medical community had been buried so deeply they could only be found by searching for an exact quote. One piece had been drastically changed to completely distort findings of the original article. Thankfully, I had printed many of the articles and saved others as screen shots. I'd learned the necessity of that the hard way, when I could no longer find a particular article I'd wanted to double-check.

It is my hope that you will feel compelled to tell others what you learn in the following pages. It may be the most valuable information that you share from this book.

Disclaimer

I am *NOT* a doctor or scientist, and I write from my personal education, extensive research, experience, and wisdom, wisdom acquired through the Bible and revelation from my Lord and Savior. None of the statements in this book has been evaluated by the FDA. This book does not claim, nor is it intended, to diagnose, treat, cure, or prevent any type of disease. The information provided is intended for your general knowledge only and is not a substitute for a physician's medical advice or treatment for any specific medical condition. Always seek the advice of your doctor or other qualified health care professional and institution with anything regarding a medical condition. Never disregard medical advice or delay in seeking it because of

---

[60] https://www.glidden.healthcare/

something you read in this book.

My goal in writing is that you move forward with more complete information, not dismiss or ignore any information.

With that in mind, let's delve into understanding a bit of the science of behind the two approaches to addressing cancer: natural health and conventional medicine.

The Natural Health Approach to Fighting Cancer

Do you recall the example of an athlete with a knee injury? We compared that athlete to someone who never exercises and both needing the same exact surgery. If everything is equal in terms of the surgeon and rehab, the athlete would have the best odds of the quickest, most complete healing because his body is already conditioned to heal. Conditioned how? As an athlete, he already:

- ingests good foods/nutrients, which feeds the cells, heals and builds the immune system (imperative!), and reduces toxin intake (compared to eating junk food).
- drinks a lot of good quality water, which helps deliver nutrients and oxygen to the cells and helps clean out toxins and the lymph system.
- exercises, which relieves stress, strengthens the immune system, pumps fresh oxygen to the cells, and causes the body to sweat out toxins and clean out the lymph system.
- gets enough rest, which is a key time for the immune system to heal the body since the body isn't devoting its resources to keeping the body in motion.

The five elements that the athlete's and our body need to create and maintain a healthier cellular environment are 1) nutritious food, 2) good quality water, 3) clean air, 4) exercise, and 5) rest. I know that comes as no surprise— it's a common-sense approach to good health, and we've heard it for years. But it's time to start implementing. Though we don't need to become athletes, we should make choices that move us in that direction. We need to get in—and stay in—good shape and good health, starting now. These five are foundational to avoiding most diseases, including cancer. They are also foundational to healing from disease.

They are counterpoint to a weakened immune system, toxins, improper diet, and oxygen deprivation, the general causes of cancer. They create an environment resistant to microbes causing an issue.

This natural health approach isn't easy in a society conditioned to take-a-pill solutions, but making lifestyle changes to improve our physical well-being and quality of life can ward off future illnesses. Thankfully there is a trend toward healthier eating and lifestyles, and many who make changes say they soon feel better than they have in years.

So, nutritious food, good quality water, clean air, exercise, and rest are the first step in healing. Let's look at a few points in more detail to gain vital insight.

Nutritious Food

You've likely heard that good nutrition while fighting cancer means we should, at the very least, eat a diet high in vegetables (especially cruciferous vegetables like kale, broccoli, and cabbage) and maintain a healthy weight. A diet high in vegetables is a great place to start.

However, it's difficult to get all the vitamins and minerals we need through diet alone, so supplementation is often required. The quality of vitamins and supplements range from useless (not absorbed and eliminated intact) to high quality and making a significant impact. The key is whether our bodies can break them down and absorb the nutrients. I recommend whole-food-based supplementation rather than synthetic nutrients.

And personally, I am a huge fan of AHCC mushroom extract, as previously mentioned.

Just as we need to consume nutritious food, we also need to understand what we are doing to feed the cancer at the cellular level and eliminate it. Cancer loves sugar. As previously described, during PET scans radioactive glucose (sugar) is injected, and since cancer cells love sugar they go into a feeding frenzy. We need to significantly reduce sugar from our diet. But artificial sweeteners are *not* the answer, in my opinion, as many cause cancer. Take time to research nature-based sweeteners for yourself. One I suggest investigating is monk fruit, since it appears to have antioxidant, anticancer, and antidiabetic properties.[61]

Let's look at food quality based on recent seed-development and farming practices. Much has been written about organic versus nonorganic foods and GMOs, and I'd like to address them briefly here. These are my viewpoints,

---

[61] https://www.healthline.com/nutrition/monk-fruit-sweetener

based on my education and research. When I research, I look for the science and facts (not opinions) and the motives of those who write the content (whether or not they are driving opinion and profit over health).

Organic products have strict standards about the seeds and all the farming processes allowed, to label a product as being organic. So, they tend to be more expensive. I think of organics as the least contaminated by toxins. (Some companies have made false claims about being organic, so due diligence is required.)

Nonorganic is conventionally grown and uses synthetic chemical fertilizers, pesticides, herbicides, and other continual inputs to increase crop yield. Although the government approves of the substances used, many consumers are becoming increasingly worried about the effects of ingesting all these chemicals.

Research online "dirty dozen and clean fifteen" for a list of nonorganic foods that are safe to eat, and which foods should only be consumed when grown organically.

GMOs, genetically modified organisms, are where the genetic material has been artificially manipulated in a laboratory through genetic engineering. Scientists create combinations using plants, animals, bacteria, and virus genes to try to improve yield or resistance to a variety of issues that could cause damage to the crop.

Debate rages on the benefits versus the health concerns of ingesting GMOs. Please take a few minutes to watch *Jeffrey Smith: Why Are GMOs Are Bad?*[62]

The most controversial example is Monsanto's genetically modified (GM) seeds that resist its own herbicide product, the glyphosate-based Roundup. Thus, the farmer can apply Roundup and the crop will not be impacted by the weed killer. However, as weeds become resistant to it, more needs to be applied, and farmers are now dealing with superweeds. Dow Chemical is introducing a new line of seeds that some are calling Agent Orange crops, to withstand even more toxic herbicides. Agent Orange was used to defoliate the jungles in Vietnam, and many veterans from that war have dealt with or are dealing with the health issues caused by that poison.

(Are you noticing how these companies that create chemical poisons are also developing seeds that will become our food?)

It seems that big agriculture, like big pharma, keeps pushing the boundaries and putting profits before safety. Please do yourself a favor and check out GMO Facts[63] by The Non-GMO Project, and do your research. Many countries around

---

[62] https://thetruthaboutcancer.com/why-are-gmos-bad-video/

the world will not accept U.S. seeds or agricultural products if they are genetically modified, and there are some extremely scary combinations undergoing testing.

Nobody knows the long-term effects of ingesting these Frankenscience products. Did you know, "Scientists have for the first time shown it's possible to create human-animal hybrids using existing genetic editing techniques"?[64] The scientists, companies, and media want us to believe the developments are positive, but what are the long-term repercussions?

If we want to reduce our odds of getting cancer, avoiding GMOs is one of the first places to start regarding food choices. Research online "Which foods are genetically modified in the U.S.?" to view a list of foods to avoid. That includes avoiding their derivatives.

Good Quality Water

I've used this phrase a few times. What does it mean?

Earlier I shared that I invested in Enagic's Kangen Water for Jerry and me, an ionic water system that changes the properties of water to make it more alkaline. This is important since cancer can't live in an oxygen-rich/alkaline-rich environment. (At first he wouldn't bother to research it, so for a time he continued to consume his favorite beverages: coffee, iced tea, and beer, which are all acidic.)

City water contains chemicals that cause cancer, so that should be avoided, even for cooking. Many bottled waters are either somewhat filtered city water or water that's had many or all the healthy properties removed. It's essentially dead water.

Spring water is oxygen-rich and helps return your body and cells to an alkaline-rich environment. This also helps improve your immune system. There are so many variables in water sources and quality that I encourage you to do your research locally.

Note that community water systems are required to deliver an annual drinking water quality report to their customers. Personally, I would recommend investing in a high-quality filtration system, or preferably an Enagic Kangen ionic water system.

Detox to Help Heal Your Immune System

---

63 https://www.nongmoproject.org/gmo-facts/

64 https://www.newshub.co.nz/home/world/2017/01/frankenscience-pig-human-hybrids-made-in-the-lab.html

Since we are generally filled with toxins, detoxing should be our very next step, after starting to correct our lifestyle choices. A primary strategy in natural healing of any given disease is to get rid of the toxins throughout our body. Often this means focusing on one area at a time (cleansing or detoxing our colon, liver, kidneys, or other part of the body).

Imagine that a bucket of swamp water represents the toxins in our body. We can try to eliminate the putrid water gradually, but it will take a long time to rid the body of toxins. It would be far better and faster if we could dump the bucket and pour in fresh water.

Essentially that's the concept of cleanses and detoxes—get rid of the junk quickly so our body can function optimally. (Drinking plenty of good quality water plays an important role in flushing out toxins.)

Cleanses and detoxing can have side effects, such as headaches, digestive issues, and feeling like you have the flu. So you will want to do your research and integrate a highly rated program (health food stores are staffed with certified professionals who can advise you) or find a natural health practitioner who can walk you back to health.

There are many ways we can detox, but regular liver and colon cleanses should be two of our first. Think of it as having a fresh filter and a clean pipe so that everything can process and flow smoothly and freely.

Fewer toxins means less of a drain on your immune system. Your immune system needs to be healthy to be free to target and kill cancer cells (apoptosis). Detoxing can help super-charge your immune system.

Smoking reduces the delivery of oxygen to the cells, creating oxygen deprivation and causing cancer, as Nobel Prize winner Otto Warburg described nearly eighty years ago. It also adds toxins to the body that cause cancer. Find a way that works for you to quit smoking, and then detox your body.

Cancer-Elimination Protocols

As you implement the above, you'll become more like the athlete and build a cellular and systemic environment conditioned to heal and maintain good health.

So, how does a natural-health approach address the disease, cancer, itself?

According to Cancer Tutor, there are three major ways to attack and eliminate cancer.

1. Safely target and kill the cancer cells.

2. Kill the microbes inside the cancer cells so the cancer cells revert to normal cells.
3. Kill the microbes that are causing the immune system to be weak (this includes the microbes in the organs and bloodstream).

Which one protocol works best on a specific cancer? You'll need to research the type of cancer and the protocols recommended, then decide based on that information.

There are over eighty types of cancer listed at Cancer Tutor and fourteen protocols, including the Budwig Diet, Cellect-Budwig, Bob Beck, Bill Henderson, Kelly Metabolic, and Rife-Beck, to name a few.

When our story resumes shortly, you'll see what the cancer journey was like with the protocol Jerry and I chose after his bone marrow transplant was cancelled.

The Conventional Medical Approach to Fighting Cancer

Now let's consider how conventional treatment addresses cancer.

Chemo, radiation, surgery.

First let's take a look at surgery.

Surgery

I have mixed reactions. I understand cutting out a tumor, to remove it from the body. It makes sense. It may also help psychologically to know that it's gone.

In the past there was a concern that surgery may cause cancer to spread. With the technology available today, doctors have a much better handle on the location of the cancer and margins around the cancer that need to be removed.

But doesn't it make sense that, if someone is having surgery to cut cancer out, it is essential to make lifestyle changes to improve the immune system and strengthen the body's ability to minimize the potential for recurrence?

Technology can be great, but there's also the potential for abuse. Research has found that the BRCA1 or BRCA2 gene is the most common cause of hereditary breast cancer. While that knowledge can be extremely helpful, women diagnosed with the gene, even at a very young age, are choosing to proactively have both breasts removed.

I understand the fear and desire to remove anything that has the potential to cause cancer, but I wonder how the surgeons can be sure they are removing all potential for cancer. I know women who have had mastectomies, only to have breast cancer appear on the chest wall, on the same side, years later.

Thanks to the natural health approach, we understand that a strong immune system and living a healthy lifestyle can fight cancer. With that in mind, I'd like to know, *Just how can cutting off a breast, or both breasts, improve the immune system?*

Recently I met three women who had areas of breast cancer cut out, only to have cancer grow back in that same breast within a few years. They were never told about nutrition and other options available to improve their health, and they had no understanding about the science of cancer.

One final note worth mentioning is that 70 to 80 percent of your immune system is situated in your digestive tract,[65] so surgery to remove cancer in that area may be seriously detrimental to your overall health. A large percentage of our population is dealing with digestive issues. They already have compromised immune systems and less than stellar health. If you want to fix your health, start with your gut (specifically, what you put into it through diet). Gut health literally affects your entire body."[66]

Radiation

What about radiation? How does it work?

Radiation therapy kills cancer cells by damaging their DNA (the molecules inside cells that carry genetic information and pass it from one generation to the next). The cancer cells whose DNA is damaged beyond repair stop dividing or die. When the damaged cells die, they are broken down and eliminated by the body's natural processes.[67] While killing the cancer cells this way sounds great in principle, radiation can also damage healthy, normal cells. Cancer is intimately related to the accumulation of DNA damage and repair failures,[68] which can lead to new or recurring cancer and other difficult long-term side effects.

I found that my initial research tended to minimize the effects of radiation. Reactions to radiation therapy often start during the second or third week of treatment and may last for several weeks after the final treatment. The primary issue associated with radiation is fatigue—feeling tired or exhausted almost all

---

[65] https://www.health24.com/Medical/Flu/Preventing-flu/your-gut-is-the-cornerstone-of-your-immune-system-20160318
[66] https://www.ecowatch.com/how-good-gut-health-can-boost-your-immune-system-1882013643.html
[67] https://www.cancer.gov/about-cancer/treatment/types/radiation-therapy/radiation-fact-sheet
[68] https://www.ncbi.nlm.nih.gov/pmc/articles/PMC3168783/

the time. Some may experience mild to severe skin problems including dryness, itching, blistering, or peeling, which will usually disappear a few weeks after treatment has finished. Skin damage can become a serious problem, necessitating a change in the treatment plan.

Other side effects may depend on the location of the radiation therapy. (Jerry experienced radiation burns on his esophagus that impacted his ability to eat, drink, and even swallow his own spit. He was also hospitalized with radiation pneumonia weeks after completing radiation treatment.)

In addition, radiation can have long-term side effects, which may include hair loss, blocked drainage that causes lymphedema (swelling), and other issues, which may continue to arise over time.

About half of all cancer patients receive some type of radiation therapy during their treatment.

In 2019, as I was skimming though an ad for the local hospital regarding hyperbaric oxygen therapy, purported to help heal certain side effects of radiation, I read the following statement. Of course, it prompted me to research further. "Serious radiation-related complications developed months or years after radiation treatment are rare. However, they will affect up to 15 percent of long-term survivors who received radiation therapy."[69]

Seriously? They consider 15 percent, about one out of seven cancer patients, rare?

So, what are some of those side effects of radiation therapy?[70] They include:

- hypothyroidism (under-functioning thyroid)
- radiation-induced pulmonary fibrosis syndrome (permanent scarring of the lungs caused by radiation pneumonia)
- heart disease
- secondary cancers
- blood cancers (including MDS)
- solid tumors
- cognitive problems
- weakening of the bones, muscles, joints, nerves, ligaments
- dry mouth, dental decay
- dry eyes, cataracts
- bowel and bladder dysfunction
- sexual dysfunction

[69] https://clinicaltrials.gov/ct2/show/NCT02425215
[70] https://www.verywellhealth.com/long-term-side-effects-of-radiation-therapy-2249293

- infertility

During my initial research on radiation, late tissue radiation injury (LTRI) never appeared. But now that the medical community has a new tool to treat the issue, hyperbaric chambers, it seems they are more than willing to be candid about all the side effects that might arise from radiation in order to market their new treatment.

Chemotherapy

And what about chemo? Chemotherapy is poison, plain and simple, and so I will keep my overview simple as well.

Considered a biohazardous material, chemo requires special procedures for handling and for cleaning up a spill. According to a chemotherapy spill kit, "Contaminated pads/toweling, the outer pair of gloves, and shoe covers are placed in the first chemo waste disposal bag, which is then knotted and placed in the second waste disposal bag. The remaining protective clothing and gloves are placed in the second chemo waste bag. Goggles can be reprocessed and are bagged separately in a zip-lock bag and sent to pharmacy with the chemo spill kit after they are removed. The chemo waste bags must be sealed securely and disposed of in the biohazard waste containers. A 'Medication Incident Report' must be filled out after any chemotherapy spill."[71]

This sounds like it'll bring good health to people more effectively than nature-based approaches? I wonder, Just how and where do hospitals dispose of these biohazardous wastes?

I'm still shaking my head that the FDA allows this, that they've approved it as the number-one treatment to be ingested (chemo pills), injected (chemo shots), and infused (chemo IV) for cancer. Personally, I can hardly believe that the FDA allows it and that we allow them to do it to us.

Okay, coming back to understanding chemotherapy. (I want to reiterate that this is extremely simplified.) Basically, cancer cells have gone rogue and are characterized by uncontrolled and rapid cell division. Many forms of chemo target cells as they divide, and so cancer cells are killed off in massive quantities. As the cells die, they release their toxins (exhaust from the car analogy), which makes the patient sick.

We often hear how quickly a tumor shrinks in size. That's from the massive die-off of cancer cells, as well as fast-growing normal cells, which causes the following common side effects.

---

[71] https://thecancerexchange.com/chemospill/

- **Digestive Tract:** As chemo kills the targeted cancer cells, it may also kill normal cells of the digestive tract. The wastes from the mass die-off overwhelm our system, causing nausea, vomiting, diarrhea, and/or constipation.[72]
- **Hair Follicles:** When chemo kills the cells in the roots of our hair, hair falls out. This may impact hair over the entire body.
- **Bone Marrow:** When chemo suppresses production of red and white blood cells and platelets, it results in anemia, fatigue, the inability to fight infection, and it jeopardizes clotting.

Because chemo doesn't differentiate between healthy, normal cells and cancer cells, it takes a huge toll on a person's health. Most notably, chemotherapy damages our immune system, which is designed to keep us healthy.

Now, honestly, how can our body fight cancer when we weaken or destroy our immune system?

Also consider this. "Cancer is caused by changes (mutations) to the DNA within cells. The DNA inside a cell is packaged into many individual genes, each of which contains a set of instructions telling the cell what functions to perform, as well as how to grow and divide. Errors in the instructions can cause the cell to stop its normal function and may allow a cell to become cancerous," according to Mayo Clinic.[73]

Since chemotherapy and radiation damage DNA—not only in cancer cells, but in healthy cells as well—how then can "normal cells grow back and be 'healthy' "?

In Short, The Natural Health Approach versus the Conventional Medical Approach

At present, one out of two men will be diagnosed with cancer, and one of three women. We are indoctrinated to believe the only course of treatment is chemo, radiation, and/or surgery. But we do have options. Conduct your own research. At least know what you think—and why—to make an educated decision regarding the many treatment options available.

Let's try to draw it all together, comparing conventional treatment versus a natural approach.

---

[72] https://training.seer.cancer.gov/treatment/chemotherapy/sideeffects.html
[73] https://www.mayoclinic.org/diseases-conditions/cancer/symptoms-cause/syc-20370588

In essence, the conventional approach—chemotherapy, radiation, and surgery—does a poor job of targeting cancer cells and does a worse job of killing the microbes. Conventional treatment kills healthy cells and can damage organs and the lymph system. Furthermore, chemo and radiation damage our immune system—the body's defense system against all illness and disease. Chemo and radiation additionally damage DNA, which may lead to new cancer.[74]

So, is it any wonder that cancer returns?

By comparison, the focus of natural health, as I've described, is to improve our immune system. We eliminate toxins and those things causing illness and disease, while giving our body all the nutrients and other things it needs to rebuild and grow strong. Then we can stave off illness and disease, including cancer, through a robust immune system, and in the process, feel more energized.

To wrap up, I'll describe the differences between Jerry's cancer treatments in a visual way, because it's helpful to envision the contrast.

Because Jerry experienced all the facets of conventional treatment, I compare that portion of his odyssey to the movie *Rocky*. It's like being in the training gym with Rocky Balboa. It's dark, it's dirty, it stinks, and you're getting the mess beaten out of you. You feel like a victim as you continue to be hammered by the effects of the chemo, radiation, and surgery. It consumes you, not only physically, but mentally, emotionally, and financially as well.

Our experience with natural health (which you'll read about in the next chapters), by comparison, felt like a walk in a meadow on a beautiful, sunny day with a calm breeze. We became light of heart once again and filled with optimism. Once we personally engaged in Jerry's healing, we were empowered.

Because Jerry had no conventional medical options left after the bone marrow transplant was canceled, he had no choice but alternative therapies. And the more we researched the new options, the more hopeful and inspired we became. We fervently pursued the natural health care plan.

Together, we had a lot of fun as we came together to make the changes in our diets and self-care. Often it felt like we were on an adventure as *we* made decisions to create the environment for healing.

Thus, it was much easier for Jerry and me to keep our focus, hope, and peace.

For us the difference between the conventional and the alternative approaches was like night and day.

Now back to our story.

---

[74] https://www.cancerresearchuk.org/about-cancer/what-is-cancer/genes-dna-and-cancer

Part 2
The Natural Health Experience

Chapter 14

Cancers Four and Five: Holistic Therapy

Jerry and I didn't post at CaringBridge unless we had news to report. On June 22, 2011, what we had to share was exhilarating. We decided to be done with oncology and to attack Jerry's blood and lung cancers naturally . . . and in the beautiful country of Spain!

And the Plan Is!!—Journal entry by JERRY HUSSEY—*6/22/2011*

We have been accepted at the Budwig Center in Málaga, Spain and will begin treatment on July 18, 2011. We will be back home August 9.

The clinic runs a twenty-day program, including weekends. No time for sightseeing other than Sunday. The rest of the time we will be learning how to eat healthy, experiencing various therapies, and the like. Included in the cost of the treatment is an apartment for twenty days.

The clinic is on the southern coast of Spain in the Costa del Sol region and not far from Gibraltar. The town is the birthplace of Picasso, so maybe this old country boy can get some culture. We are staying a couple of extra days and calling it our fortieth anniversary, a year early.

The clinic provides Wi-Fi, and we will have our computer, so we will be able to keep CaringBridge up-to-date throughout the ordeal.

As always, we ask for your prayers and support.

God bless you all, and thank you for your comments. They mean a lot to us.

The Battle Plan—Journal entry by JERRY HUSSEY—6/29/2011

Today I begin the removal of cancer from my body. I started the regimen prescribed by the Budwig Center and will be taking a boatload of enzymes, spirulina, vitamin D3, Essential Supplement (That is the name of a supplement from the naturopath)*, lemon juice, and specifically for the tumor, apoptosis and MSM (methylsulfonylmethane) supplements. This is along with the muesli of cottage cheese, flax seed, flax seed oil, and flavor enhancers such as nuts, cocoa, cayenne pepper, and limited options of fruit.*

I go to the doc for a blood test next Wednesday, and I will be extremely interested to know how my blood work compares to that of June 16. I think Dr. PM is going to be surprised. I feel great, except for my heel, and have gone back to work and making sales calls. I love my job, and it makes me happy to be with my customers.

You are probably asking, "What about the heel?" I managed to get Achilles tendinitis on June 20. I didn't do anything out of the norm, but it happened. Wednesday I couldn't walk at all and had to crawl/slide everywhere. Picture that, a sixty-one-year-old man crawling up stairs and across the floor and sliding down the stairs. My med tech daughter said it was probably tendonitis and told me to go to the real doctor. I went and was told it was tendonitis and to wrap it and stay off it for a while.

One of Diane's friends recommended I take 1000 mg of magnesium and 500 mg of calcium per day, and it would aid in healing. I started that Sunday, and . . . Tuesday I was still on crutches but walking flat-footed. . . . Today, I was down to one crutch, and tomorrow I'll keep them with me, just in case, but I think I'll be walking unaided—maybe walking like Chester on the TV show Gunsmoke *("Wait for me, Mr. Dillon"), but at least walking.*

We thank you all for your comments, your thoughts, and your prayers. Our faith in God has not been swayed. We believe He has healed me and now we just have to get the illness out of my body.

*Thank you all for your thoughts and prayers for my friend Rich. He and his family are on the way home tomorrow from Dr. Burzynski's Clinic in Houston, having been deemed cancer free. He will undergo treatment at home to keep the cancer away, and we wish him and the rest of the family all the best in his continuing battle. Our battles will continue, but we **will** win.* (As a reminder, Rich had had pancreatic cancer.)

God bless you all!

Something Is Happening—*Journal entry by* JERRY HUSSEY—*7/4/2011*

When I was first diagnosed with myelodysplastic syndrome (MDS), I was advised that if I did nothing, I would have about six months to live. If I underwent the suggested chemotherapy, I would have up to two and a half years to live.

I am beginning my seventh month of "doing nothing" medically, and I still feel good. According to my wife and friends, I look pretty good, for an old man! I do believe scalar energy—I started wearing a pendant in mid-March—slowed the decline of my platelets and prevented the need for platelet transfusions.

After the bone marrow transplant was denied due to a tumor, I believe God was telling us there was a better way. Since leaving modern medicine for alternative treatment, we have laughed a lot and enjoyed experimenting with healthy meals. I have been on the Budwig Diet since June 17, 2011, and now am on a pretty full regimen of alternative therapies. I will undergo more extensive therapies when we get to Spain on the eighteenth of July.

I thank the Lord for the direction our lives have taken, and I trust in Him to heal my body so I can live to serve Him.

Thanks for all your prayers and thoughts. I cherish you, my friends, and look forward to your notes of encouragement.

Something IS Happening—*Journal entry by* JERRY HUSSEY—*7/9/2011*

I went to have blood work and cancer markers done on Wednesday, July 6. . . .

Although there are not many changes in the blood if you look at the CBC (complete blood count), there are some positives in the components of the white blood count. . . . In short, the Budwig Diet is enhancing my immune system. . . .

I've only been on the Budwig Diet for three weeks, and I've only had their enzymes and supplements for a week. Diane and I are excited about what we are seeing in such a short time. Now we cannot wait to get to Spain and take part in the rest of the treatment. As we've said before, God put this path in front of us. If we believe and trust in Him, I will be healed. I believe the healing process has begun. Thank You, Lord!

Journal entry by DIANE HUSSEY—*7/9/2011*

I just have to say thanks for all the great messages you all post. It certainly does brighten our spirits!

Shopping continues to be an interesting adventure—it takes a lot of time to read all the ingredients on packaged items to find acceptable food. Some things you would think are good, are not so good for you, even though organic. I think we looked at every cheese before finding one made with raw milk.

(I've learned so much in the last seven years, I can't believe I was even looking for packaged foods!)

Yesterday we tried to figure out how many lemons Jerry needed for the week. We bought three dozen, but I'm not sure we bought enough. He's up to drinking the juice of six lemons in the morning and increases by half a lemon every day (I think until he gets to ten), and then decreases by half per day. It's just one of his many protocols.

(Lemons are alkaline when digested, not acidic, and cancer cannot live in an alkaline environment.)

*I am so happy and encouraged that he is willing and eager to make so many radical changes in such a short time frame. The results we're seeing affirm that the diet, supplements, protocols, **and prayers** are working!*

Thanks to everyone for the prayers. We have an awesome God who has an amazing plan. We may not understand it at the time, but it is all good!

On July 11, a major storm hit our area. We were without power for four days. I gave away the food in our refrigerator and freezer or threw it out. So, when Jerry and I came home from work, we had little to eat. We did our best to follow the Budwig Diet, but it was extremely compromised. However, we enjoyed our time together bumping comically around the house packing for our trip, with candles and flashlights for light. I love how we always became our best during adverse conditions.

Jerry and I even headed to the laundromat together to do our laundry—the first time we'd had to do that in more than thirty-five years!

I also had a little time to reflect. For years, Jerry and I'd had different interests and activities. Jerry still traveled a lot with his job, while my focus was on growing in my relationship with God and starting a natural health business. In many ways we had drifted apart.

But now we were going to Spain, just the two of us. Even the air around us seemed to crackle with excitement. After all the cancer disappointments, the worst being that the stem cell transplant had fallen through, we eagerly anticipated going to Spain and to getting his cancer *cured.*

It was bringing us together. God was bringing us together.

The power came on the evening before we left for Spain, so we didn't have to finish packing by lantern light or candles. Instead our home was bright that night, in a way that seemed prophetic.

□

We arrived in SPAIN!

Jerry and I were truly blessed to have the resources to be able to go to the Budwig Center in Málaga, Spain, for alternative treatment for his cancer. Not everyone can afford to do so. (Visit the center's website[75] and download the free *Budwig Guide* for more information.)

To keep all the treatment details to a reasonable length, here is a list of treatments and therapies Jerry received. Most therapies were done at the center, although he had homework, which he did in the apartment.

Therapies in the Clinic

Bach Flowers	IVs
Chi Therapy	Massage
Colon Hydrotherapy	Nutrition
EFT (emotional freedom technique)	Papimi - NanoPulse Therapy
Foot Detox	Power Plate
Hyperthermia	Reflexology
Inhalation Therapy/Essential Oils	SCIO-Energy Assessment

Therapies Done "at Home" (in the apartment)

Coffee Enema	Supplements
Far Infrared Sauna	Ultimate Liver Cleanse (Detox)
Iodine Painting	Nutritional Meals, Juicing

Jerry had *numerous* supplements to take. He'd always hated to take pills and often gagged. But he got better at it knowing that it was helping.

---

75 https://www.budwigcenter.com/

We felt light-hearted and enjoyed each day—what a different way to do cancer! When we blogged, we wanted to convey our excitement, hope, and adventures. We weren't writing a book then. We were sharing our life with family and friends.

I share it with you now, the alternative cancer option we chose, as well as the joy and beauty of being in Spain.

We chose life. We chose our attitude. We chose to be equipped with new information and a new approach. And we chose God.

"I have set before you life and death, blessings and curses. Now choose life." (Deuteronomy 30:19 NIV).

Journal entry by DIANE HUSSEY—*7/18/2011*

We arrived in Málaga yesterday and spent the night in a beautiful hotel downtown. We arrived at the Budwig Center today, got settled into our apartment, and went in for the consultation this morning. Jerry had a reflexology session while I learned to cook.

NO COOKING IN OIL—not even to sauté.

(We learned that all cooking oils, except coconut oil, when heated to high temperatures are carcinogenic.)

They prepared lunch for us—fish in a tomato sauce with rice, and the nutritionist also made us fresh granola.

The clinic is closed for siesta at two o'clock, so it was back to the apartment (our home for the next three weeks) to take inventory of what we needed from the grocery store.

Here's the biggest challenge so far: trying to shop for healthy/organic foods, with no ability to read/speak Spanish! The supermarket is just a couple of blocks away, and the farmers market is just one block from home. The farmers market was a haven of (super!) *fresh fish (we are less than a mile from the Mediterranean), fruits, and vegetables, but of course didn't have everything we needed.*

We got back to the apartment in time to make some of Jerry's favorite muesli (all the ingredients for this staple of the program were supplied by the clinic), *then off to the clinic for his first of ten hyperthermia sessions (every other day). Cancer can't live in high temperatures, so the goal for this therapy is to kill cancer cells and shrink the tumor in his lung. This is just one of the many therapies Jerry will receive.*

(Hyperthermia therapy was available in Spain eight years ago. It's now *finally being used in clinical trials in the U.S.)*

Jerry was able to get the Internet working. He's sleeping, and I'm heading to bed shortly as well.

I want to assure everyone that this natural health choice is a blessing. Jerry/we have been through traditional/conventional treatments three times, and this is by far the better way. God says in the Word that He has provided on Earth all that we need, and that is the premise of most of the therapies used here at the Budwig Center.

So far, we have met people from England, Canada, Florida, and New Zealand. They have all been here about two weeks, and all agree this is the best decision they could have made.

I get to participate in some of the therapies as well, and I'm taking notes. I pray that the knowledge we receive here at the Budwig Center will be a blessing to many others who choose to approach their health in positive ways, rather than through the poisons (chemo), burning (radiation), or cutting (surgery) that is practiced in the U.S. That treatment seems barbaric in light of the natural alternatives found in holistic treatments.

I mean, honestly, how many people do you know who are treating their cancer and consider it a vacation?

God's peace, and thank you all for the prayers! They ARE working!

To give you a better idea of what muesli is, the basic recipe for Budwig muesli calls for the following.

Recipe for Budwig Muesli

6 Tablespoons organic low-fat cottage cheese

3 Tablespoons flaxseed oil

2 Tablespoons freshly ground flaxseeds (they become rancid after twenty minutes)

Additional ingredients may be added for variety and taste— organic cocoa, vanilla flavored liquid stevia, ground walnuts, almonds, coconut, cayenne pepper, berries, and more. For complete directions, visit https://budwigcenter.com/dr-budwig-milk-flaxsees-oil-cottage-cheese-recipe.[76]

---

[76] https://budwigcenter.com/dr-budwig-milk-flaxsees-oil-cottage-cheese-recipe

Journal entry by DIANE HUSSEY—7/19/2011

We get to the clinic about ten in the morning, and it's pretty much nonstop while we're there with the therapies-of-the-day.

The nutritionist made us creamy buckwheat, and for dessert a healthy ice cream (of sorts). Chocolate, of course.

We also had another consult with Lloyd Jenkins PhD, naturopathic practitioner. He loaded Jerry down with more supplements. He's up to forty-five supplements a day plus other stuff—hardly leaves room for food!

You may be wondering what and why all the supplements and therapies? Essentially, cancer cells are low-energy cells. Part of the therapy is targeting/killing the cancer. Another part is making the body more alkaline (cancer cannot live in an alkaline environment). Another part is increasing the energy of the cells.

And another part is focused on relieving stress, education about nutrition and lifestyle changes, and eliminating the wastes and toxins.

It is really affirming all I learned in classes earlier this year as I was certified as a Natural Health Counselor, and I hope to bring the information home and educate people on prevention and alternatives to the traditional Western (conventional) medical treatments.

On a lighter note, they SERIOUSLY do NOT know how to lay out a grocery store. Every shopping excursion is an adventure. They certainly don't have some of staples we rely on, and they have VERY limited selections!

Searching for Kleenex was challenging. First you look down the aisle to see what the sign says. Of course, you can't read Spanish. So, you look at what's at the end of the aisle where you're standing. Unfortunately, that doesn't mean anything in the aisle has ANY correlation to what you're standing near. Paper products are not all in one place. They're scattered all over the store.

In my wandering I did find a Spanish/English dictionary. Jerry's app on his iPhone doesn't always work. I know—makes no sense that we didn't get a translation dictionary before arriving here.

We are finding that it's hard to fit eating into the day, especially around the pill-taking schedule. Breakfast is muesli, light lunch at the clinic from the nutrition lessons I get, and then we try to eat a good dinner. Tonight we had an omelet and a salad.

We're both pretty tired, but confident that this is all working as it is supposed to.

All the people in the Budwig Center are very friendly and helpful. Another couple arrived today and got the tour. Life is GOOD!

Always remember, no matter what is going on in your life, look for the good, look for the lesson, find something to be thankful for, and enjoy your journey!

As always, Trusting in God,

Diane

Journal entry by JERRY HUSSEY—7/19/2011

So far this trip has been fantastic, and the education is amazing.

As Diane said, I am going through many different therapies, from detoxification, to electro stimulation of the cancer area to increase energy, to hyperthermia to cook the cancer. It is so interesting and makes so much sense when we learn about cancer.

Treatment Day Three—Journal entry by DIANE HUSSEY—7/20/2011

Tonight it seems important to me that I include this tidbit—the goal of the Budwig Center. I underlined what spoke to us from their Wellness Cancer Guide.

"At our cancer center our approach teaches you how to 'win the battle' against cancer in the shortest reasonable time possible by implementing a multifaceted, totally natural, time-tested anti-cancer program."[77]

It IS an intense program. One of Jerry's biggest challenges is to get all the food, supplements, and therapies done every day. But we WILL win the battle—it's important that everyone understands the power of positive thinking, faith, and belief!

We had a great day! It's hard to believe all that we accomplish in one day. We went to the farmers market, then Jerry had many therapies, plus a consultation on emotional stress. The doctor found out that Jerry's pretty laid back, but stress is a HUGE factor in causing cancer. How are you doing in that department?

---

[77] *Budwig Center Wellness Cancer Guide,* July 2011. http://www.budwigcenter.com/

We both had a foot detox. The pictures are really disgusting! It is typical of what all the patients and their spouses have found in their detox sessions.

I was able to demonstrate my scalar energy pendant to the doctor today. With just one test, he was blown away and bought eight pendants. He clearly understands the value of energy in healing and keeping healthy! I am ecstatic that he was receptive to hearing about something new. So many doctors in the U.S. are resistant to listening to anyone who has something out-of-the-box to share with them!

One of the great opportunities I have while Jerry is in therapy is learning how to "cook" and prepare healthier foods. Today for lunch we made a salad with fresh almond dressing. It was exceptionally good.

The other day we were told not to cook in oil, use water instead. I made an omelet without oil last night, and tonight I made an awesome fish dish. No recipes, just adding healthy ingredients! It was really delicious (almost broke my arm patting myself on my back)!

The adventure continues! Life is GOOD!

Relaxing Day—Journal entry by DIANE HUSSEY—7/21/2011

Jerry had a VERY relaxing day today. This was the first day we seemed to really get a handle on the routine.

I thought I'd get a couple of loads of laundry done today—a couple because the washer is extremely small. I looked up all the words on the washing machine, but some don't exist in my translation book, Jerry's iPhone, or online. What is flot?

So I'm not sure if I got too much soap in it or if the machine isn't working, but eight hours later we still don't have the first load done! Jerry tried rinsing the clothes in the shower and we put them back in the washer, but it just continues to run and run. Tomorrow we'll ask for help.

We've had a lot of laughs about it, and I have a picture of Jerry sitting in front of it watching it like a little kid.

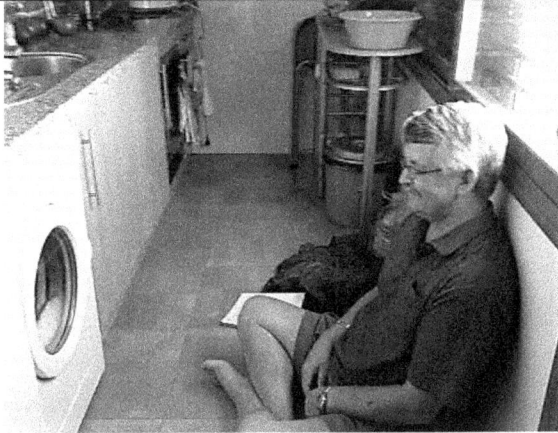

We went for a walk this evening—a bit too far. But we made it back to the apartment just like homing pigeons. :)

Jerry surprised the doctor when, during the EFT (emotional freedom technique therapy) session, he told doc that he's the happiest he's been in a long time. We really hope that this cancer journey will help many who are facing the battle to give some time and attention to seeking alternative cancer options.

Until tomorrow, resting in God's loving arms.

Thoughts—Journal entry by JERRY HUSSEY—7/21/2011

Recapping and Comparing

I think I should make some observations concerning conventional treatment of cancer and what is being done here in Málaga, since we have been here for a week.

I went through 60 doses of chemotherapy, all via IV and most taking four hours to administer. Yes, chemotherapy beat testicular cancer, but the results are myelodysplastic syndrome (MDS), caused by one of the chemotherapies. (According to current research, MDS is listed as a possible side effect with three of the chemotherapies Jerry received and also the combination of radiation and certain chemotherapies.)

Another side effect of chemotherapy is nerve damage. I now wear hearing aids, and it possibly further damaged my left femoral artery. That is what Diane was referring to about walking too far. I cannot walk very far and can hardly walk uphill.

I also underwent 51 CT scans, 28 radiation treatments, and an untold number of chest x-rays. There is a cancer tumor in my left lung that may be from all the radiation exposure. CT scans are proven to cause cancer.[78] *(X-rays can cause cancer too.)*[79]

My immune system has been pretty well destroyed thanks to chemotherapy, and I now use an electric razor for fear of nicking myself and the nick becoming infected. Your immune system is the first line of defense against cancer, and chemotherapy destroys it.

Along with chemotherapy drugs, your daily dosage includes anti-nausea medicine and whatever else may be needed to make it bearable. One of my chemotherapies was so dangerous that the nurse would stay with me for the first fifteen minutes to make sure I didn't go into respiratory arrest.

That particular treatment was preceded and succeeded by three days of steroids to help hide the pain. I'm here to tell you it didn't work. The only way I found I could rest was partially reclined in a Lay-Z-Boy. (Honestly, I know many who recount far more traumatic accounts of their chemotherapy experiences than we have. It breaks my heart every time I hear of someone being diagnosed with cancer who is starting, or who has started, chemo and/or radiation.)

Here at the Budwig Center, they focus on restoring the immune system, and detoxification is a main aspect of that. You should see some of the garbage that comes out of our feet during that portion of detox.

This weekend I undergo a "deep liver and gallbladder cleanse." It will cause me to pass whatever gallstones I may have, painlessly and completely, and the cleanse is all natural! I know a couple of people that may have been saved from surgery had they undertaken this thirty-six-hour cleanse.

Coffee enemas are another way to cleanse the liver, and once the liver is detoxified it requires a monthly enema to remain free. I used to love to drink coffee, but it is very acidic, and cancer thrives in an acid environment. The liver filters most things you ingest, so it only makes sense to clean it occasionally. With chemotherapy, the liver takes considerable abuse. Under the Budwig plan, I have chosen to join Diane in making many dramatic lifestyle changes for the betterment of my body. Coffee enemas are but one small part of the change.[80]

---

[78] https://www.naturalnews.com/032120_CT_scans_cancer.html
[79] https://www.cancer.org/cancer/cancer-causes/radiation-exposure/x-rays-gamma-rays/do-xrays-and-gamma-rays-cause-cancer.html
[80] DISCLAIMER: This is provided for informational purposes only. Please consult your physician before doing a liver cleanse. Cleanses were done under the direction of Jerry's naturopathic and integrative doctors.

If my experiences dealing with cancer over the last eleven years can cause only one person to consider alternative, non-invasive medicine, then maybe my journey has been worth it. I have a feeling in my soul that cancer was defeated yesterday and now I'm on the road to recovery. We will continue to address my other ailments, like hearing and walking, and pray that God will heal those also.

This center is focused on God's natural healing, and you can certainly feel His presence.

Thank you for your prayers and continued support. It means a lot to us. God bless!

Treatment Day Five—Journal entry by DIANE HUSSEY—7/22/2011

WOW—the days are flying by! Two couples leave to go home over the weekend. One returns to Florida and the other to England. It really is amazing how close we all became in a short time.

The couple from Florida are Baptist, and the couple from England are Muslim. "Mike" from Florida was on his knees praying for the Muslim woman, while I was saying good-bye to the Muslim man. As I usually do, I reached out to give him a hug. Earlier in the week he told us that he doesn't hug anyone other than his wife. I started to back off, but he reached out and gave me a hug. Barriers get broken down when we are going through issues together. We all exchanged e-mails and got pictures. It has been a really wonderful week.

I can't even remember all the therapies Jerry got today, including a few new ones. They sure keep him hopping.

Lunch was fabulous—a layered fruit cake, all healthy.

As for our issues with the washing machine . . . One of the staff members came over and pushed the same buttons on the washing machine that I did—except that it worked for her. Then Jerry did the next load while I went to the market, so that will be Jerry's job. He's doing all the laundry and hanging it to dry on the rack.

We have an awesome breeze coming in the windows—no screens, almost no bugs. It is beautiful here! I hear it is very hot at home and over most of the U.S.

Wishing you all peace and God's blessings!

Saturday—Journal entry by JERRY HUSSEY—7/23/2011

We've had an interesting Saturday. Fun, and at times laughable. Diane and I WALKED to the beach ("Just a little further," she kept saying—it has to be at least a mile) and found that the sand is gray in color and there are a lot of stones. The Mediterranean is colder than you would imagine. We decided that a lot of the people on the beach should not wear bikinis and speedos, even in their secret bedroom closets.

I get to stay really close to the toilet tonight and tomorrow, due to the onset of my deep liver cleanse. It will clear my body of gall stones, and a periodic cleanse will prevent gallstones from forming. A clean liver is a happy liver!

(At the bottom of a recent page, I noted a disclaimer about liver cleanses. I kept that information in the journal entry because it's one of the most difficult protocols Jerry experienced in natural health, but it's virtually nothing compared to his experiences with chemotherapy and radiation.)

To begin the cleanse, I had a cup of 50/50 orange juice and grapefruit juice mixed with two tablespoons of oral Epsom salts.

I think I'll let Diane finish this. I must excuse myself and retire to the reading room!

Journal entry continued by DIANE

Jerry just had his second OJ/grapefruit/Epsom salt cocktail. At 11:45 he'll have another one, except that it will include some lemon juice and a cup of olive oil (ugh).

It seems a lot of my time is spent in the kitchen. Today we both made the fresh OJ and grapefruit juice. It was fun. Jerry didn't get underfoot too much as he finished our laundry.

I went to the market again today—twice. I forgot to take my dictionary and had to go back to get it!

Life's an adventure. Enjoy it!

Whew! It Is Over!—Journal entry by JERRY HUSSEY—7/24/2011

If you read yesterday's post, you know that I began the ultimate liver cleanse. I finished it today and can tell you the cleanse does work.

After a rather uneventful night (only one trip to the bathroom) I experienced anticipated results this morning. I passed many stones with the largest being about the size of a pencil eraser. As promised, the passing of the stones was completely painless. By doing this cleanse every six months or so, I should never have to go through gallstones and surgery. The inconvenience of having to stay around the house for eighteen hours is minor in comparison.

It's Sunday. Diane went out for a walk and to see if any stores were open on Sunday. I asked her to look around for a used bookstore where we might find a paperback in English. We will see what she finds. She took along her English/Spanish dictionary just in case.

Chapter 15
Spain—Week Two!

Monday, Starting Week Two—Journal entry by DIANE HUSSEY—*7/25/2011*

We are becoming the veterans. Today was the last day for the Canadian couple, so more good-byes. He is healing his stomach cancer; his wife has dementia. The clinic recommends that the patient bring a support person, family member or friend, to help with meal preparation, shopping, errands, and the like. Imagine trying to do it all yourself while you have cancer and having to take care of someone else at the same time in a foreign land.

We had several new patients (will become friends) arrive over the weekend—a Spanish couple (the wife speaks pretty good English), a man from Holland with his friend, and a couple who live in Portugal.

So as veterans, we help the newbies as much as we are able.

We went to the market and I set off the alarm as I was going in as well as coming out. I didn't get frisked and they didn't make me empty my bag or fanny pack. Maybe it's my magnetic personality? :)

Jerry's treatment continues to go well. We have a personal sauna in our room. Jerry decided I should go first. You get wrapped into it like a mummy, with a towel to lie on and a towel over you. It heats up to 122 degrees F and you lie there and sweat.

It was great. Sweating is actually very good for you. It eliminates toxins very well. I felt really energized and decided to walk the courtyard for exercise before showering.

I met the guys from Holland while walking. They were on their way back from the clinic and hadn't had dinner, so I gave them our leftovers. Neither are comfortable in the kitchen, so I promised to take them to the farmers market and help them with their food.

We really like where we are living. The apartment building uses motion detectors for lighting in the hallways. I think the motion detectors on our floor recognize us now, so they are not alarmed when we get off the elevator. We have to wave at them to get them to turn on. I guess they want us to be neighborly and wave! :)

Keep smiling. Enjoy your journey. Be a blessing!

Tuesday, Week Two—Journal entry by JERRY HUSSEY—7/26/2011

Another new patient arrived today, with his brother and sister-in-law for support, so the clinic is getting very busy. We are settled into our routine and try to show the new kids the ropes.

(Many of the patients are very sickly and weak when they arrive. Often patients or their families resort to holistic health clinics, like the Budwig Center, after being told there's nothing else the medical community can offer. They search for an alternative with a strong resolve to beat cancer, or out of fear and desperation. Natural health tends to be an option of last resort. I pray that people start to consider it as their first option.)

The new patient, a gentleman living in Portugal, was told the hospice program in that country is not good, and that he should return to his home country where they have better treatment. But he and his wife are people of faith and were not willing to accept hospice (their perception is that hospice is a death sentence). So, like the rest of us who found the Budwig Center, they chose to combine faith and holistic health measures in looking for a cure.

As Jerry and I both learned in our research, very often alternative medicine does what conventional medicine doesn't—it heals! It's just too bad that so many people have been weakened by surgery, chemo, or radiation before coming here.

I'd like to ask you to pray for Eric, one of our new friends from Holland. He doesn't know the Lord, and he is scared. He has two small children, ages two and five. He is not sleeping or eating well. He has a LOT of pain.

The people who have a relationship with God, Jesus, or Allah, as we saw with the Muslims here last week, seem much more peaceful.

With all the cancer stories we're hearing, from all the different countries, we pray that you will seriously look at your life, and the lives of your loved ones, and consider the changes you can make to improve your health.

Getting enough rest is one of the keys, so I'm signing off for now.
God bless.

Halfway!—Journal entry by D<small>IANE</small> H<small>USSEY</small>*—7/27/2011*

It is truly hard to believe Jerry's halfway through his twenty-day treatment already! Today the last of our original group left to go back to New Zealand. Mary has an amazing attitude and is always a breath of fresh air and a blessing to all. She will be missed, but we WILL stay in touch.

I continue to read and reread the Budwig Center Wellness Cancer Guide. *It is truly amazing how many therapies Jerry has access to, how they work to kill the cancer, detox, build the immune system, and give the body what it needs. We cannot stress enough that THIS is the way to go! The education is invaluable, the therapy regimen SO much more patient-friendly than the conventional treatments in the U.S. (as well as many other countries, as we are learning).*

We don't seem to have the interesting challenges we had, like the washing machine or setting off the alarms at the market. Except yesterday I set off the alarm going in and coming out. Finally security checked my bag. The Spanish/English dictionary that I had purchased there had a bar code inside that I was supposed to remove. Thankfully I had put the receipt in the book so "no problemo." (Practicing my Spanish.)

I went for a walk this evening and found the most beautiful park in the historic district. We hope to spend an afternoon in the park on Sunday. Friday afternoon and Saturday, we plan to take a tour bus around Málaga so we can plan our final weeks' forays. We have settled into a comfortable, peaceful routine now and really love southern Spain. What an incredible health treatment and vacation rolled into one.

We hope you are . . . considering ways to help yourselves and others improve your health and future.

Blessings!

Kitchen Duty—Journal entry by D<small>IANE</small> H<small>USSEY</small>*—7/28/2011*

After we got back from the clinic, and each had siesta in the sauna, we started juicing. Vegetable juice provides all kinds of nutrients needed to fight cancer among MANY other benefits.

It is kind of a big deal: washing all the vegetables in hydrogen peroxide to kill any salmonella, bacteria, or e-coli; rinsing them; cutting; and juicing. Jerry helped, and we had a lot of fun.

What all did we put into it? Carrots, beets, spinach, cucumber, celery, green pepper, zucchini, and some other greens—maybe swiss chard?

*Fruit juice is **not** recommended. Too much sugar, and cancer LOVES sugar. It feeds on it. Eliminate all refined sugars as much as possible from your diet!*

We decided to make a liter of the vegetable juice so we'd have it for the next couple of days. We'd make a bit and taste it. A few of our comments: Tastes too green. It's tolerable. It tastes like dirt. Let's put some Celtic sea salt into it before drinking.

When you're eating to live instead of living to eat, somehow you can eat and drink things that don't taste so good, knowing that they are going to be beneficial.

The sauna we use in our apartment is nothing like you would imagine. It looks like a silver, space-age sleeping bag with Velcro. (We owe you some pictures on this one.) We turn it on for 50 min (previously we were doing 40, and we're working our way up to 60), turn it to 50 degrees C (122 degrees F), and we just lie there sweating, usually going to sleep.

Personally, I wake up VERY refreshed. It is detoxing us. Although we sweat and soak the towels we are wrapped in, the sweat is different. I know it sounds peculiar, but it feels like a dry sweat—it evaporates quickly—and I don't feel sticky from it.

And usually I have a song running through my head after the sauna, James Brown's "I Feel Good."

Hope you're feeling good too! (Now you're going to have that song running through your head.) :)

Friday, Week Two—Journal entry by DIANE HUSSEY—7/29/2011

Jerry had a light day at the clinic. I did almost as many therapies as he did. We both had a foot detox, and the water was MUCH clearer than the first time we did it. Jerry has had four of those treatments. I've had two. I guess the personal saunas and all the other things we've been doing are working!

After lunch (lentil soup), Jerry went back to the apartment. One couple asked me to stay and pray for them. The husband is extremely weak and frail. They are an incredibly sweet couple. He was a priest and missionary in Africa for many years, and she had been a nun. They met after both had left their ministries. I'm looking forward to hearing more of their stories next week when he is stronger. Please be praying for him. His name is Wim, and he was originally from Holland.

We went on the tour bus for a ninety-minute tour around the city. Málaga is a beautiful city with a long history.

Jerry had kind of a tough day today. He didn't get enough sleep and just couldn't get going.

Also, the group we had in the clinic last week was a much closer-knit and spiritual group than this week's group. The staff is great, the naturopath and integrative doctor are wonderful, but it was really good last week to have others to share with.

This week, however, the patients seem to have far more serious and advanced cancers. The waiting area has been fairly empty, whereas last week it was always bustling.

Tomorrow is a new day, and we will spend the day touring, trying to find something healthy to eat, and trying to remember to take all the supplements!

VACATION DAY!—Journal entry by DIANE HUSSEY—7/30/2011

Today was a day of vacation. We rode up to the fort/castle at the top of the mountain. Jerry's energy levels are pretty low, so I ran around taking pictures, since the trails and stairs are pretty steep.

We also did a bit of shopping—bought the T-shirt, as they say. We also found a new market with a healthier selection of grocery items, and blueberries! Jerry's been missing them in his muesli.

Before leaving the U.S., we decided to use this trip in part to celebrate our fortieth anniversary a year early. So today we bought a bottle of Málaga wine. It is a red wine but VERY sweet. (Just like Jerry!)

I'd like to request specific prayers: that you would pray for his red blood cells to increase in numbers and size, and that his hemoglobin would increase. I'm sure that will help his stamina. The rest of him is really quite good!

Thanks so much for the prayers. (I'm posting his picture. He looks pretty darn good, doesn't he?)

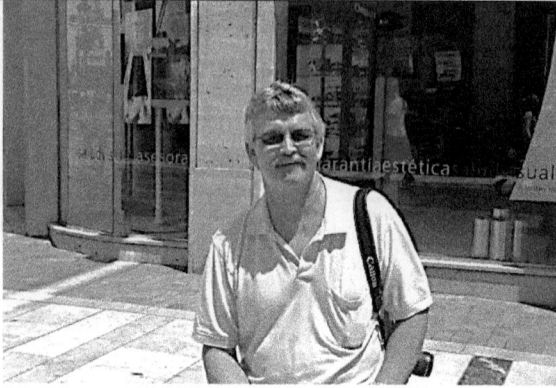

Loving LIFE!!!!! Praying you're doing the same!

Sunday, a Day of Rest—Journal entry by D̲IANE̲ H̲USSEY̲*—7/31/2011*

And we certainly did rest today. Jerry only did a little laundry, and I took the sheets and towels to the roof to hang them on the clotheslines they have installed up there for the residents.

One of our friends from Holland was also doing laundry. The friend he came to support had been taking sixteen painkillers a day when he arrived. His therapies started Monday. On Tuesday he'd wanted to leave, but the friend talked him into staying. He is now on ONE painkiller a day!

We went to lunch at a vegetarian restaurant. We are always excited that the cab drivers can figure out where we want to go. Jerry had a lasagna with a Spanish flair, and it was quite good. I had a ravioli that was excellent. Somehow the waiter managed to understand me when I told him I wanted to take my leftovers with me. People at the next table were laughing as I tried to explain myself. They were quite tickled when I got the next phrase right: Foto por favor.

Jerry's energy levels continue to be low, maybe because he's getting a bit homesick. Our apartment is nice, but small, and we've never lived in a bustling city like Málaga.

Also, I know it is weighing on his mind, how will he be able to travel and do his job while trying to eat his Budwig muesli, continue with his dietary restrictions, and keep up with the timing of his protocols and supplements. He loves his job and really doesn't want to retire. It will all get worked out, I'm sure.

He hasn't been sleeping well. Tonight he had some Celtic sea salt, it's

supposed to help, before going to bed. We'll see if it works.
   God's peace.

Chapter 16
Spain—Week Three!

Monday, Week Three—Journal entry by DIANE HUSSEY—8/1/2011

We can't say enough about the staff here—very good, very caring, and they will do whatever they can for you. While here, you get what you need. Period. You pay one set fee, and if you need something, they give it to you, just like that.

Jerry mentioned how tired he'd been over the weekend, so he got an IV with iron. It helped him with the energy he's been lacking.

We're staying a couple extra days after his treatment is done. They don't have anyone coming in, so we get to stay in the apartment the extra nights free of charge. Is that wonderful or what? We are VERY thankful that we were led here. It's an amazing experience!

Spain goes on holiday for three weeks in August. The group that came in the week after us is the last group until September. We feel very fortunate (blessed!) that we were able to get in when we did!

Today I had a session of EFT—emotional freedom technique. It really is freeing of emotions, stress, and tension. Jerry also found it extremely helpful.

(EFT is a practical and useful application, and you can look in up online. However, for me, prayer, time with Jesus, and the Bible give me even more peace and freedom.)

I bought the coconut I needed to make raw chocolate, and my almonds are soaking. If I get up early enough, I may get it made and in the freezer before going to the clinic.

Recipe for Raw Chocolate

1 cup of almonds or cashews
8 dates, stones removed (be sure there is no sugar added as a preservative)
½ cup of cold-pressed olive oil

Soak nuts overnight in water. Drain. Blend nuts, dates, and olive oil well in a food processor. Then add:

¾ cup of shredded coconut
⅓ cup of raw chocolate powder

Mix well and put in the freezer overnight before serving.[81]

I want to thank all who prayed for our friend from Holland. Jerry reminded me that I had asked for prayers for him. He's the one I mentioned yesterday who had gone from sixteen pain pills/day to one/day in less than a week. The power of prayer, coupled with doctors who use their God-given talents, have yielded some spectacular results.

*Our body has an amazing ability to **restore itself** via holistic modalities and revolutionary technologies. Hyperthermia, Papimi - NanoPulse Therapy, reflexology, Chi Machine, Power Plate, foot detox, and far infrared saunas have widespread use in Europe, but may not be readily available in the U.S.*

(Some alternative therapies used in Spain are finding their way into the U.S. medical system, but generally aren't a focus of conventional cancer treatment here. They are normally found in natural health practices— nutrition, supplements, detoxing, massage, EFT, colon hydrotherapy, and more.)

By eliminating toxins and adding God-supplied natural foods, herbs, vitamins, and supplements, we CAN transform our health!

Life is GOOD!!! Keep the faith!

---

[81] From our July, 2011, copy of the *Budwig Center Wellness Cancer Guide.* Used with permission.

Journal entry by DIANE HUSSEY—*8/2/2011*

It was our first day that I can say we felt a bit challenged and a tad upset. Jerry has been having more problems with the circulation in his feet and legs. They have been cramping, going numb, and the coloring is a bit on the pale side.

He asked one of the staff members to interpret some questions for the Spanish doctor and was told she'd be there in fifteen minutes. The staff member forgot to come back to Jerry, and the clinic closed for siesta. We had to go back to the apartment and return to the clinic a couple hours later for hyperthermia. Jerry was frustrated knowing that we wouldn't have an interpreter when we got to the clinic, and therefore wouldn't have any answers.

The doctor and nurse could tell something was bothering Jerry, and I tried to explain, but the language barrier got in the way.

I had my trusty little Spanish/Ingles dictionary and was trying to look up all the appropriate words: leg, feet, cramping, numb, or anything else I could think of, but I didn't have time to find all the words.

The basic question was whether Jerry's problem with his feet and legs was related to anemia (a red blood cell or hemoglobin issue, resulting in deficiency of oxygen) or a circulation problem. As I'm trying to figure out what to say and how to say it to a nurse and doctor, I can't state it nearly so succinctly. I mean, how do you act out "anemia/deficiency of oxygen or circulation problem?"

So here we all are, trying to translate for each other. Jerry can't hear very well and has real trouble understanding them, so I'm translating what I understand they're saying, they're talking/translating what I'm saying, and we have a great game of charades going. :)

Incredibly, we pieced it all together that his legs and feet were going numb, his energy was low, and his foot color was not right—they were white (blanco).

Somehow, when I explained femoral-to-femoral bypass, she was able to understand the question. Was this a vascular problem or anemia?

She explained it is a vascular issue, and when we come home Jerry will probably be visiting a vascular surgeon. The doctor who did his surgery ten years ago had said his femoral-to-femoral bypass would last approximately two to five years. Jerry said the doctor would probably be amazed that he's still alive.

So, although it was a bit more challenging than previous days, we did manage to find the humor in the situation and were able to laugh about it in the end.

Tomorrow is a new day, a bright and cheerful day, in sunny southern Spain. We hope yours is just as wonderful!

Always Hope—*Journal entry by* DIANE HUSSEY—*8/3/2011*

There is always hope! We had affirmation of that twice today.

First affirmation: Yesterday our minds reverted to what we knew about Jerry's circulation problem and what had been done previously with Western (conventional) medicine. So that's what we thought would have to happen again when we returned to the U.S.

But Jerry received homeopathy and other treatments today, which seem to have helped! He received a shot in each hip near the femoral bypass. Immediately he felt it down to his toes in his right leg. The left not so much, but that is the worst of the two. He is scheduled to have it done again before we leave. I think they used Liquid Plumber or Drano to unclog the blockage. :)

He also had magnet therapy, some manual manipulation, and I'm not sure what all, to stimulate the circulation. Tomorrow he will get cayenne pepper capsules. Cayenne pepper is a great stimulant for poor circulation.

So, we are believing that he is healed by natural means and believing with the faith of a mustard seed that he is receiving what is needed according to the Bible. We are standing in faith and praying for healing in Jesus' Name and according to the Word!

Second affirmation there is always hope: I want to close with an amazing story about one of the patients who came in last week. He was misdiagnosed by the medical doctors and was in terrible shape. He was the one I'd prayed for and mentioned in Friday's post, Wim. He was unable to eat more than two tablespoons of food without pain. His systems were shutting down, and basically, he just had skin covering his skeleton. He was so weak that they were bringing him his treatments to his room (their apartment is within the clinic).

He had a very difficult weekend, but the cancer is disappearing from his body.

His wife and the doctors could feel the tumors in his abdomen before, but the swelling and size of the tumors has gone down tremendously. They can hardly feel the tumors anymore!!!

Now he is able to eat one-fourth of a papaya, has been able to eat fish, fruit, most of a serving of muesli (six tablespoons), not all at once, but is eating quite often all day.

His pain has subsided tremendously, his spirits have been raised, and it is a miracle, according to him and his wife.

MANY people are praying for healing for Wim.

What made the difference—prayer, or all the treatments and protocols by the doctors?

Give credit where credit is due.

Jesus is the Great Healer, and I perceive that the doctors allow God to work through them, to guide them in their treatments. They have the knowledge and discernment to promote and accelerate healing.

We are seeing and experiencing amazing healing results all around. We believe.

We are both available if you know someone who is facing the cancer battle and wants information about alternatives or doesn't quite know which way to turn. Remember, Jerry has had it all: the poison (chemo), burning (radiation), and cutting (surgery), so he knows what he's talking about. Been around the block, as it were.

Feel free to share this blog with others. We hope that Jerry's journey will prove beneficial to others!

LIVING AND LOVING!

Thursday, Week Three—Journal entry by DIANE HUSSEY—8/4/2011

It is hard to believe we've been here almost three weeks. We have learned so much, seen so much, and want to share it all with others. I keep reading prayer requests on Facebook and in e-mails about this person with this type of cancer, another with a different type of cancer, and I just want to reach out to them and help.

Mentally I think we're both ready to come home. It will be easier to prepare our foods with all the utensils I have at home, food processor, American measurements, and a better variety of pan and bowl sizes. It will be easier shopping as well. We have a limited selection here, and it really is hard to shop for a specific diet when you can't read ingredients. (What was I thinking? We had the freshest of fish and vegetables right around the corner!)

I added some pictures today. You've got to love their sense of humor over here. They always refer to whether something is on this side of the river or the other side. Well the river pictures are posted. In fact, the volleyball game and soccer/volleyball courts are IN the river!

(The "river" is only a river during the rainy season. While we were there, it was just a trickle that I could have stepped over. I spent a fair amount of time one evening watching a soccer/volleyball game that was being played "in the river." As in soccer, the use of hands is forbidden, and it was incredible to watch how they were able to play and control the ball with just their feet, thighs, chests, and heads.)

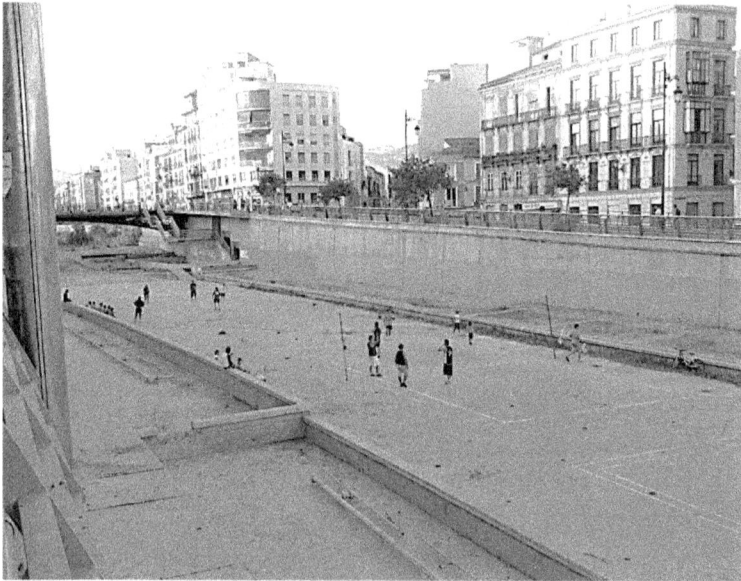

Málaga is a beautiful city, and I'm enjoying my evening walks. We are near enough the Central Historical District that I can walk there. I wish Jerry was able to join me. . . . Someday—we're believing!

Keep smiling! It's good for the soul!

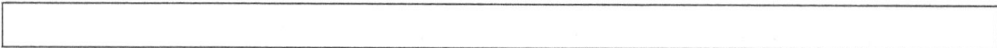

Friday, Week Three—Journal entry by DIANE HUSSEY—8/5/2011

We are rounding the final turn and coming into the home stretch. Jerry had some of his final therapies today, but still has some more left on Monday.

His exit Quantum Test showed a marked improvement in some areas. A few areas were excellent when we arrived and still are. One area went down—his overall energy level.

We cannot say enough about this place. The clinic was so busy they weren't able to get a blood draw on Jerry, so they made an appointment at a clinical lab. They called for a taxi and gave us the money for the cab fare and blood draw. They wrote down the addresses for the cab drivers to get us there and back. We came to this clinic and they said all procedures were covered, and they meant it. Whatever extra Jerry has needed they've done it.

Honestly, these people and this clinic are fabulous! (FYI—The blood draw cost $17.61. Can anyone tell us how much a blood draw is in the U.S.? I will have to check our insurance records when we get home. How much does Medicare pay? Just curious.)

Tonight there was some kind of festival going on downtown in the historic district. I talked to one of the vendors, and he said they'd be there again tomorrow. I will go back down to see everything in the light.

It doesn't get dark here until almost 10:00, and I often leave to go for my walk around 8:00. Here lately I've been getting back to the apartment around 10:30. I'm just fascinated by the city and the people.

(When we first arrived, I wasn't sure how safe it would be to go walking through the city, but the longer we stayed, the more comfortable I felt. Jerry needed a lot of rest, and usually went to bed about the time I left to go on my walks, so I wasn't abandoning him. The following day he enjoyed hearing about all that I'd seen. I needed the refreshment of exercise to keep my energy and spirits up and flowing, and my exploits energized Jerry.)

Jerry is going to rest this weekend. I will be going out to get lots of pictures to share with him. Some of the therapies he gets are pretty powerful, so he may just need more time to rest and relax. We push pretty hard during the week.

Jerry is missing a big multi-class reunion this weekend and sure wishes he could be there. He is there with you all in spirit and promises that we will be there next year! Please take lots of pictures and videos!

God bless!

Saturday, Week Three, A Day of Opposites—Journal entry by DIANE HUSSEY—8/6/2011

Today Jerry stayed in the apartment and rested. He sorted pictures of our trip, played on the computer, and napped.

I did the sightseeing we had planned and took LOTS of pictures. I took the tour bus to the fort and took pictures from all aspects, then walked down the mountain, taking more pictures. I walked all afternoon and into the evening, stopping for dinner at a sidewalk restaurant. I was gone all day.

Tomorrow two more areas I want to experience—the park and the beach. Then a trial packing to make sure everything fits.

Good night, and sweet dreams!

As I'm reading, it almost seems like I'm selfish—going off on adventures through the city and leaving Jerry in the apartment alone. I was doing what we had wanted to do together, but couldn't, and he encouraged me to go. I took pictures so we could share what I'd seen and done. It was the best we could do with his energy levels what they were, and I am ever so thankful we were able to do it. Through most of our marriage, Jerry had been the photographer, so as I was taking pictures, I was thinking of him and the different shots and perspectives he might enjoy. Since Jerry enjoyed history, I spent extra time in the museum in the fort taking pictures of things I knew he would relish seeing. No, he probably wouldn't have taken pictures of most of those things, but it was my way of bringing the day back with me. I always loved to do things for Jerry, and in my heart and spirit, we were doing the day together. Later we were able to spend time together reviewing all that I'd seen and done through those pictures.

Getting Ready—Journal entry by DIANE HUSSEY—8/7/2011

We're starting to get ready to leave. We've packed some things, started cleaning the apartment, and mentally are making the transition. We're cleaning out the refrigerator and planning on the foods we can take on the plane. I think Jerry's a bit more ready to come home than I am. I love Málaga—never thought I'd enjoy it so much.

Jerry's energy levels continue to give us some concern. I'm hoping he gets an IV of iron tomorrow and we get the results of the blood test back so any changes can be made.

I did make it to the beach today and tried to bring some entertaining pictures back to Jerry (I'm his eyes and feet). I was also trying to be discrete while taking a few of them. I don't believe topless and toothless go together, but there she was! And God forgive me for judging people, but some people have no business going out in public NOT dressed properly!

I also stopped at the park and took lots of pictures of flowers, trees, foliage, architecture, the ship in the port, and waterpark. I tried to capture the utter beauty as well as the heart of the city. I went back this evening— Jerry thought there were going to be fireworks, and I wanted to hear whether the OOOOHs and AAAAAAHs sounded any different in Spanish. I was also hoping the lights they have strung up across the street were going to be lit, but they weren't. No fireworks, so I can't tell you about OOOOHs and AAAAHs.

Summary of the trip from my perspective. It was wonderful. We are believing that Jerry is healed of the cancers. The Budwig Center receives our endorsement.

Jerry has mostly asked/let me post, now it's HIS turn to give you all his take on the trip!

It's Time to Say Good-bye—Journal entry by JERRY HUSSEY—8/8/2011

Without question, this has been the best decision we've made concerning cancer treatment for this old body. I truly do believe the cancer is cured and now it is just following the protocols and letting my body heal. Just like surgery or a broken bone, it will take a while to heal and I will have to have a transfusion every now and then until my body is able to take care of itself. Some of the supplements I take will end soon and some will end in six months or so. Some will never end.

The dramatic part of this healing is maintaining a diet conducive to supplying my body with the foods directed by God that have His healing power. Diane is going to have a challenge in providing a diet consistent with the requirements, but she is a good cook and will do well. As I travel throughout my territory on business, it will be my challenge to stay as true as possible to my diet, and that too will be accomplished.

We were packing up yesterday and today, and Diane had a sad look on her face. She has toured all over Málaga on foot and by bus and has fallen in love with the city. I agree that it is a beautiful city, more ancient and more historic than anything you will find in the States. The people are wonderful also, even as we try to negotiate the language barrier.

 Yes, more than the medicine itself, this place is a healing center. Not only do the staff care for the patients, but the patients and their support people care for each other. A wonderful Spanish lady was sitting with her husband today while he and I were getting infused (with iron)*, and she noticed my IV had a leak at the connection. She called the nurse and had my leak fixed without hesitation. Just good people helping people, and people I will miss. I said "gracias" and she said "you're welcome."*

 I pray that none of you are diagnosed with a cancer, but if you are, please consider this place as an alternative to U.S. treatment. I do believe God stands in the entire clinic and works His miracles.

 Thank You, dear Lord, for standing with Diane and me and all of the others who have passed through this clinic.

 Many of you have commented about how great Diane is, and I've managed to keep her head from swelling—so far. She really is a wonderful person, and I'm glad to be celebrating our thirty-ninth anniversary in a little less than a month. I am blessed to have such a wonderful wife.

 God bless you all, and thank you for posting your thoughts and prayers. We have enjoyed reading the comments you've posted and have laughed at the comments from left field. Thank you all, and I hope to see you soon!

Here's the rest of the story that didn't make it into the CaringBridge journal. Remember, Jerry had blood drawn on Friday, August 5. When the test results came back Monday, August 8, the Spanish doctor had a serious look of concern on her face. Thankfully Jerry didn't see that look.

She showed me the hemoglobin numbers, but I wasn't too concerned because I didn't understand Spanish or know what all the numbers meant. Plus, I knew he'd had low numbers in the past. We continued to walk in faith and trust—believing for the best.

What is hemoglobin, and what does it do? It's the protein molecule in red blood cells that carries oxygen from the lungs to the body's tissues and returns carbon dioxide from the tissues back to the lungs. Thus, with the low hemoglobin levels, his body was starving for oxygen, and this was one of the reasons for his lack of energy.

The Spanish doctor mentioned a transfusion, but Jerry wasn't comfortable receiving blood in Spain. He wasn't sure how safe it was, recalling mad cow disease (was that only England or all of Europe?), so he called Dr. PM to set a transfusion appointment for early Wednesday morning.

While going through all Jerry's medical records, I couldn't understand much about his blood work since it was referenced in Spanish, but I could understand the word for *hemoglobin*, and he was down to 6.1. For men, the average hemoglobin levels range from 13.5 to 17.5. Generally, as I understand it, blood transfusions are given when hemoglobin falls to the 7.0 to 8.0 range.[82]

With hemoglobin half to nearly one-third the normal level, it's no wonder Jerry's energy levels were so low.

---

[82] http://www.medscape.com/viewarticle/760919

Chapter 17
"We're Home—Chaos Reigns"

We're Home—Chaos Reigns—Journal entry by DIANE HUSSEY—*8/11/2011*

We drew the line in the sand this morning and WILL get organized and on track. Since Jerry's last post:

We were awake over twenty-four hours from the time we got up to the time we got home. Yes, we managed to get in a few little naps here and there, but not much.

Jerry had wheelchair service at all the airports. What a blessing! We had a glitch at Heathrow, which caused us a bit of consternation about making our flight to O'Hare, but we made it. None of the issues were any larger than what we've all come to expect when we're flying these days. . . .

We arrived in Chicago, flew through customs (YEAH!), and my parents came to pick us up. We'd left Jerry's car at their house. They only live twenty minutes from the airport, so it works well. Jerry's car lights are not normal, and when I thought I'd turned them off, they weren't off. So we had a dead battery.

My dad got his jumper cables out, and we got it started. It showed that he had no gas, so we drove two blocks to get gas. What do you do when you get gas? Turn the car off. Uh-oh!!! But it hadn't had time to charge, so it wouldn't start. I walked home and got my dad to come over to try jumping it again, but it wouldn't start. We tried and tried with no success.

FINALLY, we got the car started (thanks to a good Samaritan with super heavy-duty jumper cables who happened to drive in at the perfect time) and found that we actually had about a half tank. The reason it showed empty was because there wasn't enough power to register the gas gauge.

It was after 11:00 p.m. when we got home, and we had to get up early to be at the doctor's office for a transfusion. I was going to drive so Jerry could rest. I guess I'd left my interior lights on when I was looking for something while packing three weeks earlier, so I also had a dead battery, and Jerry ended up driving. (He has a company car, and I'm not supposed to drive it.)

His hemoglobin was way down, so he got two units yesterday, will get one today, and may get another tomorrow. We had encouraging news that his white blood count (immune system) is improving, so that's a very good sign.

*(When his blood was drawn at the oncologist's yesterday, just five days after the last draw in Spain, his hemoglobin was down to 5.2, which is **extremely** dangerous. I read that at 5.0 the heart may stop. One of the nurses said he shouldn't be able to talk, much less walk into the office.)*

We have been researching some information on stimulating the body's ability to manufacture its own red blood cells that we learned about in Spain. We are still researching the several types available for the best option and solution and will discuss our finding with Dr. PM. He has his concerns but is working with us and not pushing Jerry into anything.

We picked up Connor (our dog) yesterday, so Jerry is very happy about having him home. We had taken him to his foster family weeks before, when Jerry was supposed to get his BMT. Jerry is VERY happy to have him back. He has really missed him.

(Animal lovers understand that unfailing and unequivocal love that knows no bounds, and yet it is nothing in comparison to God's love for us.)

So, we had another very long day yesterday. We got home about 6:30 p.m., and I immediately lay down to take a short nap. I woke up at 3:00 a.m. We had no dinner, and we really haven't had time to do much of anything since we arrived home.

Jerry has gotten way off track on taking his supplements and protocols, so we start afresh today. I must get to the store because we have virtually nothing here to eat. We had no power for four days right before we left for Spain and either took the food from the refrigerator and freezer to my parents or threw it out. So we really are starting out from scratch.

Jerry has gone off to work and then to get a transfusion. I am heading to the grocery store and then to his job to take him some lunch—making beans and rice with fresh vegetables diced to throw on just before serving.

We pray that we are able to settle into a routine in short order. We really appreciate your prayers. These past couple of days have really worn us both out.

But today is a new day. Take a deep breath, give thanks, and praise God! All will be well!

When we got home from Spain, my friend told me that she knew everything was going to be fine, because when she and her husband came over to check on our home, there were frogs everywhere—on the front door, siding, sliding glass door, planter, in the bushes, everywhere! She said, "He's really watching over you guys."

What did she mean?

Years earlier I had told her that FROG is a word that has far more meaning to me than a little green animal that hops and croaks. I had heard that the acronym stands for:

F—Fully
R—Rely
O—On
G—God

FROG has been a reminder and guiding light for me for years. We believed in God's healing powers and stood on Bible verses that called on us to trust in the Lord.

"Trust in the LORD with all your heart, and lean not on your own understanding; in all your ways submit to him, and he will make your paths straight" (Proverbs 3:5-6 NIV).

"May the God of hope fill you with all joy and peace as you trust in him, so that you may overflow with hope by the power of the Holy Spirit" (Romans 15:13 NIV).

"Cast all your anxiety on Him because He cares for you" (1 Peter 5:7 NIV).

Hopefully, you've seen how the messages in these few verses have been woven into the fabric of our story.

Sunday evening, August 14, Jerry developed shortness of breath and diarrhea. It's not uncommon to hear of healthy people getting sick after flying, and since his immune system was still low, we thought Jerry had caught a bug on the trip home. His symptoms were bad enough that we went to the emergency room. He was hospitalized for observation and released the next day.

☐

I'm at a loss to even try to convey my thoughts at this point. God had our backs, and natural health gave us hope. Were we being naïve? There is power in prayer, and we had our heads up and eyes on Jesus.

Earlier I referred to the story in the Bible about Peter being able to walk on water as long as he kept his eyes on Jesus, but when he was distracted by the wind and the waves and took his eyes off Jesus, he sank.

The story is found in Matthew 14:25-33 (NIV).

> Shortly before dawn Jesus went out to them, walking on the lake. When the disciples saw him walking on the lake, they were terrified. "It's a ghost," they said, and cried out in fear.
>
> But Jesus immediately said to them, "Take courage! It is I. Don't be afraid."
>
> "Lord, if it's you," Peter replied, "tell me to come to you on the water."
>
> "Come," he said.
>
> Then Peter got down out of the boat, walked on the water, and came toward Jesus. But when he saw the wind, he was afraid and, beginning to sink, cried out, "Lord, save me!"
>
> Immediately Jesus reached out his hand and caught him. "You of little faith," he said, "why did you doubt?"
>
> And when they climbed into the boat, the wind died down. Then those who were in the boat worshiped him, saying, "Truly you are the Son of God."

I'm fairly convinced that if we'd understood the gravity of the numbers (and if those distractions had led to doubt), we'd have sunk. I am *so* thankful that we both agreed on the course of treatment and had the same high level of faith to sustain us through these difficult times.

☐

Journal entry by DIANE HUSSEY—8/23/2011

Well, it's been a week since I posted, so I guess it's time for an update. Jerry just drove up to Wisconsin on a sales trip, just two to three days as we try out packing food, since he is still on a very restricted diet.

His immune system is still low, so no raw fruit or vegetables, unless I disinfect in my kitchen with Kangen Water. Here's the basic list of what he can't eat, so you have a clue of how difficult preparing for a trip can be.

*No meat, no dairy (except the cottage cheese in his muesli at breakfast), eggs are okay, no fried foods, no sugar, no white flour, nothing sautéed or cooked in oil unless it is coconut oil, and all foods **should** be fresh. We can only do what we can do, and we are doing the best we can.*

He has to prepare his own muesli, so he took the stick blender, coffee grinder (to grind flax seeds), a hot plate and pot to cook in, the hand juicer, dishes, a dozen lemons, black-eyed peas (two meals), pasta w/ pesto sauce (two meals), mock meat loaf, quinoa, fruit, avocadoes, hard-boiled eggs, blueberries for his muesli, fresh raw tomato sauce for his pasta, cottage cheese, flaxseed oil, and that's just for three days! He will have to be able to eat at restaurants and eat salads before he can fly anyplace!

He had a doctor's appointment yesterday. I'm a bit testy about Dr. PM. He doesn't like me doing my research. We'd heard about EPO (erythropoietin) shots in Spain and had talked to the doctor last time we were in his office about Jerry receiving those shots. It helps stimulate production of red blood cells/hemoglobin. Instead, the doctor wanted to give him Darbe. EPO is derived from human sources, and is administered once a week, while Darbe is administered twice a month, but it is derived from Chinese hamster ovaries. Yep, I just saw you raise your eyebrows! Human sources versus Chinese hamster ovaries. Which would YOU want?

So the doctor gave in when Jerry said he wanted EPO because it had worked for our friend's mother and grandson in Europe. Yeah! Victory!

I almost lost it, though, when Jerry got his shot. He had a new nurse, and neither one of us cared for her even before she gave him the shot. She said she wished she had suckers to give out for good patients like him.

"SUGAR????? REALLY? WHY WOULD YOU GIVE SUGAR TO CANCER PATIENTS?" That's outrageous, especially since she works in an oncologist's office!

"Why not?" she asked.

*"Because cancer **thrives** on sugar!" was my response.*

"No it doesn't," she said.

*ARGGGGHHH!!!! Okay, if there is one thing you learn from this cancer journey it's this—**<u>CANCER LOVES SUGAR</u>**. Doctors often prescribe a PET scan to confirm a cancer diagnosis. Radioactive glucose (sugar) is injected, and the image created on the PET scan lights up where the cancer is basically in a feeding frenzy on the sugar.*[83]

---

[83] https://beatcancer.org/blog-posts/5-reasons-cancer-and-sugar-are-best-friends/

(If you recall, Jerry's first oncologist, Dr. Blinders, encouraged him to eat a big bowl of ice cream every night to try to regain some of the weight he lost, and drink two quarts of Gatorade for electrolytes!!! ARGGGGHHH! Cancer not only loves sugar, but thrives in acidity as well, so the doctor could not have given Jerry a more terrible recommendation. Hopefully, by now, oncologists and their staffs have learned that sugar and acidity feed the cancer they are trying to kill. Oncologists also commonly recommend so-called nutrition shakes to cancer patients, and many of these shakes are packed with sugar!)

So there you have it. We continue on the journey, putting one foot in front of the other, and praying for our miracle! In addition, we love to share the cancer information that might be helpful to you, or to people you may know.

I SEE You, aka ICU—Journal entry by DIANE HUSSEY—9/7/2011

Wow—where to start? We've been extremely busy since returning from Spain. Last week our daughter, Tara, came up to visit. We had a GREAT time, lots of laughs, and it was just good to be together.

We celebrated our thirty-ninth wedding anniversary on Saturday, and Jerry's sixty-second birthday on Sunday.

Our son Devin was scheduled to come up, but he received a full scholarship for a solar program, so he had to postpone his visit—perhaps Veterans Day, or as his school schedule allows.

Brandon moved recently to Paris, Texas (where my grandfather was born—small world), so he couldn't come up either.

So life has been treating us good. Jerry has been working, really sticking to his diet, and has been taking his supplements, but we haven't been able to stay on task with detoxing. There just aren't enough hours in the day.

The past couple of days have been spent in ICU at the hospital. Shortly after Jerry woke up yesterday morning, he started coughing up blood. We went to the ER at the local hospital instead of driving the hour plus to the hospital that has all his records.

One breathing treatment was able to calm the cough, and he stopped spitting up blood. He had another chest x-ray, CT scan, and a bronchoscope. They found a blood clot in his lung and pneumonia. He is still in ICU but going a bit stir crazy—doesn't fit the profile of most in ICU. He looks great, doesn't feel sick, energy has been good.

His blood counts were low, so they gave him two units of blood, two platelet transfusions, and antibiotics. We have managed to find food on the hospital menu that he can eat, although I did take dinner up to him last night, and he is asking for homemade pesto and pasta tomorrow.

We had some issues with hospital staff who are not open to or accepting of our choice of alternative therapies, the questions and concerns we raised regarding standard operating procedures, antibiotic prescriptions, and even blood draws. Some were just offended that we would dare ask questions. Others mocked us.

(Jerry was allergic to penicillin, so they wanted to give him Levaquin. We told them, "No, because of the potential side effect of tendonitis and even rupturing of tendons." Remember, Jerry had recently been on crutches due to Achilles tendonitis? I'd learned about the side effects of Levaquin when I'd had a reaction to it a few years prior—my heart had started beating so rapidly I thought I was having a heart attack. I just love how God always seemed to prepare us!

It had become *very* hard to draw blood from Jerry, due to vein damage from chemo and all the needle sticks in his arms from blood draws, IVs, and blood transfusions. Because we were actively involved in Jerry's care and wouldn't blindly acquiesce to whatever the techs and doctors wanted to do, they copped an attitude. We tried to explain how difficult it was to get Jerry's blood, and the tech took offense and insisted she could do it. (I'm also a hard stick, so watching her stick my Jerry was traumatizing to me as well, as it is to anyone who has to endure it.) I forget how often she stuck Jerry and fished around with the needle, bound and determined to draw blood. She didn't succeed and repeatedly hurt Jerry. Finally, the phlebotomist for babies and preemies was called and used a baby needle.

Knowledge is good, but we need to be prepared to defend ourselves. One doctor had the audacity to suggest that we leave and go on to a different hospital. Because Jerry had coughed up over a cup (8 oz) of bright red blood, we were afraid he was going to hemorrhage before getting to his regular oncologist and hospital.)

Anger on our part actually was a good thing, I think. When a person makes choices about their health care, when they take the time, effort, and energy required to make informed decisions, there will come a time that they will be tested. We faced it head-on and didn't back down.

We have a right to ask questions and be involved in our own care. There are doctors who have a god complex, who bully and intimidate patients and staff. Hopefully, we were able to affect some change.

We have chosen a conservative approach for Jerry's care for several reasons. It's too long to go into here, but we believe it is the wisest course of action. That means we do not know how long he will be in the hospital.

We are asking for prayers for healing of the blood clot in his lung, as well as his body's healing. The Bible says where two or three are gathered together . . . Let us all gather together in spirit and pray for Jerry and all those who need healing.

And just so we all don't take life too seriously—check out the new picture—it made Jerry and the nurses laugh to see the smiley face I drew on Jerry's knee.

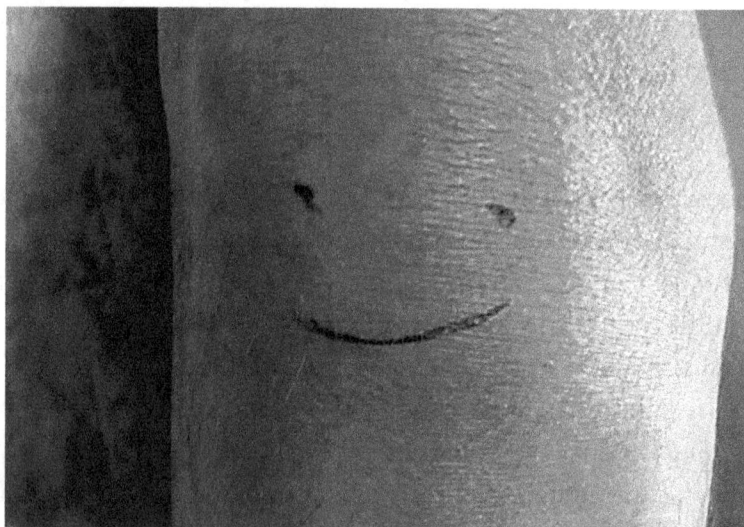

Out of ICU—Journal entry by DIANE HUSSEY—9/9/2011

Jerry was moved from ICU yesterday and is now allowed to take his supplements! We still don't know how long he will be in the hospital, but the longer they keep him, the more they will start to see alternative medicine at work. Yesterday I went to Jerry's previous hospital to pick up his last CT scan and reports and talked to Dr. PM's head nurse. I told her that I don't think Western (conventional) medicine knows how to measure Jerry, because on the surface his numbers look terrible. He truly defies the numbers reported in the blood tests. (I like to say that Jerry reflected what hope and faith look like.)

Thank you all for your prayers. We are feeling them. We had a few *challenging days, but **we are back!***

All praises and glory to God! We declare healing in the Name of Jesus, and we pray that the Holy Spirit flows through us to touch the hearts and lives of others.

Be a blessing!

So We Choose to Be Positive—Journal entry by DIANE HUSSEY—9/10/2011

Here's the latest—some good news, some not so good, and our honest feelings.

Jerry is expected to be released from the hospital Monday or Tuesday. We like the oncologists we have talked to at this hospital, which is MUCH closer to our home, so we plan on making a change.

The doctor (whom I'll call Dr. Heart, for his compassion), who gave us the diagnosis and prognosis, is candid and frank, combined with caring and compassionate. Tears welled up as he discussed his grandfather's battle with cancer, and his decision to become an oncologist.

So, we thought we'd share the bad with the good tonight. Here's a quick recap.

Jerry was diagnosed with MDS eight months ago—a pre-leukemia caused by the chemo he received ten years ago. It is usually treated with chemo, but Jerry has chosen not to go the chemo route, and at this point with his low blood counts, the chemo would kill him. Not an option.

Yesterday he was given new information. Here it is in his own words.

Journal entry continued by JERRY

I haven't coughed up blood since Tuesday and haven't had a fever, so the docs think they have the blood clot and the pneumonia under control.

The CT scan on Tuesday showed a mass 1 x 1.5 cm in the left lobe, and a blood clot and pneumonia in the right lower lobe of my lung. (We knew about the mass because that was what had kept him from the bone marrow transplant. It had grown.)

There is a suspicious shadow on the lymph nodes in the upper abdomen. Also, there are lesions on my sternum and ribs. Interestingly, these same symptoms, including the pneumonia, were present in the CT scan conducted three weeks ago when we returned from Spain. I believe my original oncologist was trying to protect me from the ominous findings since Western medicine cannot cure me.

We had a long talk with the local oncologist here (Dr. Heart), *and I told him my history and asked for his honest opinion. Until further evaluation, he said, he had to make the assumption that the lesions and mass in my lung was stage IV lung cancer (keep on smoking, folks). He said that stage IV cancer and a third occurrence is very aggressive, and stage IV is treated to prolong life, not cure. He cannot treat the lung cancer since the myelodysplastic syndrome (MDS)* (which was caused by chemo) *has destroyed my blood, and to try to treat the MDS would take longer than the life I have left, six to nine months, based on current Western medicine.*

I am taking a Neupogen shot once a day to build my white blood cells, and that seems to be working. My WBC is about normal. I am also taking a shot of EPO to help my body generate red blood cells (RBC), but I only get that weekly and have not seen any results yet, so my RBC and hemoglobin are down terribly. Those are the findings of Western medicine.

We received an e-mail from Lloyd Jenkins PhD, naturopathic practitioner, our Spanish naturopath, telling us of a product he is having great success with. This product will attack blood and bone cancers and cause the cancer to basically destroy itself. We have the product on order and will let you know the results.

Yes, Western medicine says six to nine months, but Diane and I are not accepting it. We believe that our faith in God and our association with alternative medicine will see me through. I want no sympathy, no tears, because I am positive, and I want everyone around me to be positive also. I am in no pain and don't anticipate much change in my routine once I get out of the hospital.

Journal entry continued by DIANE

As the title says, SO WE CHOOSE TO BE POSITIVE. We continue to stand in faith, believing for the miracles and trusting God at His word. We continue to remind ourselves that "nobody gets out of this world alive." So very true, and it puts kind of a light-hearted spin on a typically dark subject.

None of us is guaranteed to live through the day, the week, or the month, much less a year. We've seen and heard about people passing away suddenly from accidents, heart attacks, aneurysms, strokes, and other life-ending events.

Jerry has been given an arbitrary time frame. We choose to be proactive and get things in order, clean out, and get rid of things we don't need or want (we've been married thirty-nine years and have accumulated lots of stuff). We choose to look at the situation as if we were planning to move, and what do others need more than we do?

We are both on the same page, standing strong together, and looking optimistically toward the future. We are excited at the prospects of the new alternative cancer treatment from Spain and believe that God continues to direct our path.

We pray that our strength and courage will be contagious to our family and friends, and that your prayers and support will continue to supply the energy and healing we need during these challenging times.

We also believe that Jerry's journey will be helpful to others who may be facing similar battles, or that it may help someone you know who may need hope and encouragement.

Keeping our eyes up and on Jesus! (Because if you look down, you'll sink like Peter.)

It is now 2020, as this goes to print. Is this next post as relevant, being that it was written eight years ago? Although there is no legislation on supplements before Congress at this time, I believe it is still relevant and important.

When Jerry and I started posting the CaringBridge journal, we didn't realize that it would become a platform for the advocacy of natural health.

The following request was in response to an FDA-proposed mandate that threatened dietary supplements. In the early 1990s, when the FDA threatened something similar, the consumers staged a massive revolt, and Congress passed a law prohibiting the FDA from banning popular nutrients.

Senator Durbin's bill, introduced in July 2011, in the midst of Jerry's cancer battle, was again threatening to regulate dietary supplements, even to include many fish oil formulas and natural plant extracts. That was why we were so vocal on the overreach of the FDA over our health.

IMPORTANT REQUEST—Journal entry by DIANE HUSSEY—*9/13/2011*
  This request is not just for Jerry. It is critical for everyone who takes vitamins, supplements, or knows someone who does.

It is essential that we stand up for our rights to choose our health care options, and not have the government, big pharma, doctors, and hospitals dictating what we can and cannot do with our health care choices.

*If you have been reading this journey for any amount of time, you know that we have chosen alternative health care for many reasons. But at this point, even **if** Jerry were open to American health care, there isn't **anything** they can do for him at this point.*

Here is our request.

FIRST: If you haven't yet watched Burzynski's movie, Burzynski: Cancer Is Serious Business,[84] *please take the time. It exposes the collusion, corruption, and conspiracy between the FDA, medical societies, National Cancer Institute, and big pharma, and is critical to understanding what is at stake if we allow the FDA to take control of natural health.*

This movie was instrumental in Jerry's transition to alternative health. The lies, distortions, lack of concern regarding human life, and vindictiveness by the FDA and other agencies is well documented.

SECOND: Read the article and/or watch the video by Dr. Mercola titled "Red Alert: FDA Set to Ban Your Supplements."[85]

THIRD: Contact your congressional representatives.

FOURTH: Forward this information to others. Copy and paste into an e-mail.

The FDA/big pharma wants to control vitamins/supplements and natural health alternatives.

Are they doing a good job now with the pharmaceutical industry? How about all the fast-tracked drugs for big pharma that are now at the center of lawsuits? Have you heard the commercials for "call 1-800-BAD-DRUG"? The FDA approves of chemotherapy and radiation, which are KNOWN TO CAUSE CANCER. They approve drugs that have a litany of side effects including cancer, cardiac arrest, stroke, and death.

Dr. Mercola's article is a great summary and overview about the bill and alternative health. Reading the article, you will find that natural health products and supplements don't come close to the hazards of FDA-approved drugs.

Do you know anyone who makes a living or supplemental income representing vitamin/supplement products? The actions of the FDA have the potential of driving many small businesses out of business. Thousands upon

---

[84] https://www.youtube.com/watch?v=rBUGVkmmwbk
[85] https://worldhealth.net/forum/topic/462/

thousands swear by the results they've experienced from taking these types of products.

One final rant. The FDA wants to control what God has given to us—the plants, herbs, minerals, vitamins, and supplements. This is in stark contrast to the free license they are giving to Monsanto and other companies manufacturing genetically modified organisms (GMO). God-given or Frankenscience? Is there really any question about which is better? (My dad feeds the birds and squirrels. They refuse to eat the GMO corn.)

This is literally a fight for Jerry's life and the lives/health and well-being of many others. *That is why we are asking you to take the time to read the information, watch the movie, contact your congressional representatives, and spread the word about the FDA wanting to hijack our individual choices and access to natural and alternative health care.*

I would hope to see an uprising of all who are reading about our cancer battle. We have tried to always keep the messages positive and uplifting and give it over to God. I think all that we have asked is for prayer.

Now I'm asking that you join us in standing up in righteous anger, not only for us, but for the health and well-being of others—now and in the future. It may not be affecting you personally right now, but you just may want options in the future. If you don't stand up now, you may not have the right.

Still trusting in God! (But not trusting the men/companies/institutions who are perverted by greed, power, and control.)

Thankfully, that restrictive legislation didn't pass, and there are currently no national attempts to restrict natural and alternative health care as was attempted in 2011. We do, however, need to remain ever vigilant.

Chapter 18
Winter 2017—The Quest for Truth:
Cancer Five

Jerry and I would have liked to have been able to stay on a purely holistic course to attack his cancer, but that wasn't possible. Jerry's blood levels had been so low that transfusions were life-sustaining, and the shots to try to help his body manufacture red and white blood cells were also needed, although we weren't sure how much they actually helped.

One thing that hurts me to think about was how caught up we became in the diet, food preparations, supplements, therapies, doctor appointments, and blood transfusions. We again fell into a trap of busyness. And when we are busy, we don't seem to be able to find enough quiet time with God, the Bible, focused prayer, or time for each other.

I have wrestled over whether and how to introduce this last medical record discovery into the story.

In reviewing the CT scan of 8/15/2011, done under Dr. PM's care, I duly noted the nodule in the left lung.

On the prior study, there was a nodular density in the left upper lobe which measured approximately 0.8 x 1.1 cm. This lesion currently measures 1.1 x 1.4 cm, and has therefore increased in size since the prior study. There is also a new nodular density in the posterior right lung on series 8, image 108 measuring 1.2 x 1.5 cm. In addition, there is a hazy infiltrate in the posterior aspect of the right lower lobe, likely pneumonia.

from August 15, 2011, document (page 1)

Of course we'd known that was what had kept Jerry from the bone marrow transplant, but Dr. PM had never revealed this "new nodular density in the posterior right lung . . . measuring 1.2 x 1.5 cm" *or* the "likely pneumonia." I only discovered them while "sifting" through the medical documents years afterward, two more bombshells that struck and left me reeling.

And of course, we were never told of the existing 8 mm nodule in the right lung that the BMT team had discovered in the 6/2/2011 CT scan. They'd only mentioned the one nodule in the left lung.

Why?

Was it because we'd challenged Dr. PM about AHCC and hadn't bought into the experimental study he'd proposed? Did it fall into the pattern of nondisclosure and cover-up that seems all too prevalent in our story—another mistake and oversight? Or had he been trying to protect us?

Three weeks after the 8/15/2011 CT scan, Jerry had been admitted to our local hospital's ICU, diagnosed with pneumonia and coughing up quantities of bright red blood. We honestly had been afraid, with Jerry's low platelet levels and blood counts, to try to drive to the hospital Dr. PM was affiliated with for fear Jerry would hemorrhage and die before we got there.

Reading the CT report, I grew aggravated with Dr. PM for his lack of candor and tired of the battle of sifting for nuggets, the endless months of *sifting. Contrast. Light/dark. Truth/lies. Good/evil.* All of it. I just wanted to be done with all the searching.

That's when I saw it—something I'd overlooked several times. A simple statement and date. "Comparison: 2/7/2011."

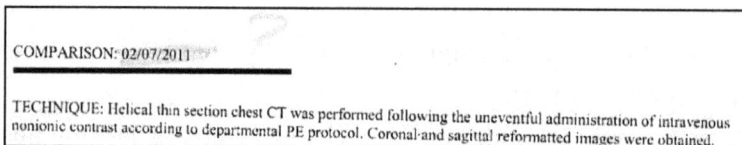

COMPARISON: 02/07/2011

TECHNIQUE: Helical thin section chest CT was performed following the uneventful administration of intravenous nonionic contrast according to departmental PE protocol. Coronal and sagittal reformatted images were obtained.

from August 15, 2011, document (page 1)

Why is this important? Because there never was a CT scan done on 2/7/2011.

Or was there?

That sent me scrambling through all the records again, every stack, page by page. Where *was* the report? Could it be lost? How would that be possible?

My mind worked in overdrive. Wait, I still had all the insurance and billing records in my tax files. The payment for the 2/7/2011 CT scan definitely would be there.

I dug those records out and methodically sorted through them, certain I would find cause to legally go after Dr. PM and the BMT doctor and hospital. For what? I wasn't sure, except that it seemed that if they'd withheld information so they could bilk us and our insurance company out of money to pay for treatment without being candid about test results, I felt there had to be something criminal there.

But I found no record. Not a single bill for 2/7/2011. No insurance payment for that date or the dates around it. *Nothing.* The only testing he'd had in February 2011 had been on February 28, which had initially revealed his therapy-related MDS.

It didn't make sense then, and it still doesn't.

Could there have been a mix-up, with someone else's record finding its way into Jerry's file? That is possible, I imagine, but the nodule is located in the left upper lobe in both scans. Is that too big of a coincidence?

After reviewing all the medical records dealing with the CT scans—nodules, their sizes and locations—and the impact a scan in January or February 2011 would have had on Jerry's treatment, this is my theory. And if it sounds like a conspiracy theory, I'm just being candid, sharing my thought processes, since I never found resolution to the supposed CT scan from 2/7/2011. I will leave it to you to decide.

Neither Dr. PM nor Dr. BMT wanted a CT scan on the nodule of 7/9/2010. Why?

HOSPITAL

DEPARTMENT OF DIAGNOSTIC RADIOLOGY

Patient Name: HUSSEY, JERRY   Age: 61 years   Sex: M
Account Number: Date of Birth:
Patient Location: CT SCAN HP

Accession #:	Procedure Name:	Exam Date	Ordering Physician:
CT-	CT Chest W/O Contrast	7/9/10 9:27:40	

Results
HISTORY: Lung cancer

COMPARISON: 01/29/2010

TECHNIQUE: Helically acquired axial images were obtained through the chest without IV contrast as per request per the ordering physician. Additional sagittal and coronal reformatted images of the chest were performed.

FINDINGS: No definite axillary, mediastinal or hilar lymphadenopathy is identified. Postoperative changes are again identified within the right upper hemithorax, with associated post radiation change as well. Probable scarring is present in the right lower hemithorax. A 3 mm nodule is present the medial aspect of the left upper lobe. No new suspicious parenchymal nodular densities or focal infiltrates are identified.

Evaluation of the unenhanced upper abdomen demonstrates decreased attenuation of the liver, suggestive of fatty infiltration.

Copies to:

Print Date: 06/06/11
Print Time: 4:02 PM   Page 1 of 2

July 9, 2010, document

While I analyzed from every angle, trying to understand why, I became extremely cynical, thinking if Jerry had MDS *plus* a secondary cancer, Dr. PM probably figured we wouldn't be open to the experimental cancer treatment he'd proposed, and that would have cost him plenty in terms of lost revenue.

"But wait! It's your opportunity to help others!"

"This experimental program is considered the best course of treatment for MDS at this time."

"Taking part . . . may or may not make your health better. . . . There is no proof of this yet."

"You or your health insurance plan will be billed."

"Develop new products."

And if Dr. BMT, who had seen all records, including the CT scan from the year prior, had done an initial, current CT scan and found that the nodule had grown and was potentially cancerous, he wouldn't have been able to bring Jerry into the bone marrow transplant system. All the appointments, tests, and procedures—potentially tens of thousands of dollars in billing—would have been lost.

Both doctors would have been impacted regarding their ability to "sell" us on the treatment they'd each wanted to do on Jerry. That could have cost them and their facilities a lot of potential revenue. Does it seem reasonable or too big a stretch to surmise that the lack of a CT scan in January or February had been marked by greed?

But what aggravates me even more, is the wondering. If someone had ordered the scan and we had known that Jerry basically had no acceptable options (in our minds) through conventional medicine, perhaps we could have started along the natural health trail sooner.

Would that have made any difference?

I have no idea. I console myself with the fact that God was ever present and knew everything as we went through it. He had a plan, and I am so thankful we avoided the BMT and were able to do cancer a much better way. God has given me the determination and documentation, and He won't let me rest until the truth about cancer is brought to light.

There is a markedly heterogeneous appearance of the sternum, likely related to metastatic disease. There is a discrete lytic lesion in the left side of the sternum, present on the prior study as well. Many of the ribs demonstrate diffuse heterogeneity suggesting diffuse bone metastases.

IMPRESSION: No evidence of pulmonary embolus. New small bilateral pleural effusions. Increased size of the nodule in the left upper lobe of the lung and interval development of a new nodular density in the right lower lobe, likely metastatic disease. There is also a mild infiltrate in the right lower lobe which may represent pneumonia.

Heterogeneous appearance of many of the bones, all likely representing bone metastases, particularly involving the sternum which appears more heterogeneous than on the prior study.

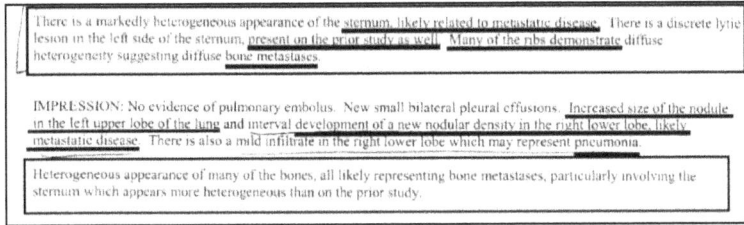

from August 15, 2011, document (page 2)

Finally, regarding the rest of the information in the 8/15/2011 CT report, Dr. PM had addressed none of the issues. He'd never mentioned the potential pneumonia, or that it appeared the cancer had metastasized to the sternum and bones—another bombshell.

Yes, we had known at this time that Jerry's MDS, the cancer caused by chemotherapy, would likely claim his life, but it now seemed crystal clear that an unwritten policy of the medical establishment was, and is, to withhold important information from the patient and his or her family, and to keep it among the medical practitioners.

That was our experience with oncologists since almost the beginning. Because of that practice, we didn't have the chance, or the choice, to be motivated to address Jerry's health much sooner, or to seek other treatment options, in a way that could potentially have saved him.

I cannot believe that our experience in this is unique. It certainly appears that millions of other cancer patients and their families aren't being told important information, just as we weren't, information that, if they were told, may spur them to seek other options and other outcomes.

Had Jerry been in the last few months of his life at the time and nothing could be done, I can actually understand that an oncologist may choose to avoid causing more stress to the patient and family, since that may be the most compassionate way all around to "do no harm."[86]

But because we had been actively involved in pursuing Jerry's healing through natural means, the lack of disclosure by Dr. PM almost seems like sabotage to me.

As that realization struck, it sent me spiraling again.

At least Dr. Heart had respected our requests and had been honest with Jerry about what appeared on the report.

Even so, I found myself thinking, *If I hadn't gone through Jerry's medical records, I never would have known!* And if God hadn't kept giving me the

---

[86] When translated, the actual wording from the Hippocratic Oath is, "I will abstain from all intentional wrong-doing and harm." https://en.wikipedia.org/wiki/Hippocratic_Oath

vision of sifting, and words of contrast, I never would have continued my quest for truth.

Chapter 19
Roller Coaster

New Protocol—Journal entry by DIANE HUSSEY—*9/27/2011*

Jerry has started the second week of his new protocol. It has been a bit challenging to get it all straight—the timing of when to take what was a bit confusing.

Packing his lunch is really quite complicated, but we are managing. Since he gets to eat honey every day, he really gets some treats, like French toast and oatmeal/apple pancakes, both served with honey and fresh fruit.

(The "new protocol" works like a Trojan horse. It combines the sugar of honey or maple syrup with alkalinity—baking soda. The cancer feeds on the sugar, but it ingests the alkalinity at the same time. Cancer cannot survive in an alkaline environment, and the alkalinity kills the microbes within the cancer cells, so this kills the cancer. Simple! Known as the Trojan Horse Protocol, also called the Jim Kelmun Protocol, this is recognized as an effective cancer option, used in conjunction with other therapies.)[87]

His spirits are good, and he worked a full day in the office today. He is still working as much as he is able. He had a couple of doctor appointments last week and received blood and platelets. That seems to be happening about every two weeks.

His foot detox was really disgusting on Sunday. I celebrate and say it attests to the cancer being killed and all the cellular debris being pulled from his system.

Today I opened Loving Health and Wellness, my business focusing on detoxing, cancer education, and living a healthier life. It is based primarily on the information we got in Spain and from my schooling as a natural health consultant.

(As of this writing, I am launching my coaching business as a cancer health coach and considering starting a crusade, to help people use natural health to win the battle against cancer. For more information, visit www.DianeBishopHussey.com.)

---

[87] https://www.cancertutor.com/kelmun/

We wish all of you good health and God's blessings, and that you will start to take good care of yourself.

Journal entry by DIANE HUSSEY—*10/4/2011*

Today Jerry received the rest of his supplements. These came from Europe, so they took just a bit longer to arrive. One is to increase cellular energy, and the other is a product called Tumor Control.

Jerry had his weekly visit with the oncologist. They took some blood and decided he needed a couple of pints plus hemoglobin, so it was off to the hospital to get filled up. We found out that the EPO shots that he's receiving cost—are you sitting down for this?—$3,000 per shot! And he gets them weekly. I think Neupogen, the shot he gets daily, is about $800. Thankfully the insurance has agreed to pay. We've met the deductible, and I'm praying there's no copay on them.

The EPO shots are to try to help stimulate his body to produce healthy red blood cells with hemoglobin and platelets. They do make his long bones ache, legs and arms, so it's not without side effects, but so far, it's not too bad.

We've had some really cold and ugly weather, so I pulled up much of my garden over the weekend. Of course, this week we are going to have bright, beautiful, sunny weather in the 70s. Well, at least we got the winter fertilizer on at the right time!

All the days seem to run together—just a blur. They start out with, What do you want for breakfast?, and then, Lunch? as I pack his cooler and he heads out to work or the doctor's office. Every day it's, "How are you feeling? How did you sleep? What's for dinner?" Virtually every night I'm making juice for the next day. Mostly the time seems to revolve around food and the supplement schedule.

Although it is best to make the juice when you're going to consume it, so it's fresh and has the most nutrients, I'm just not up to getting up early every morning to make it. Juicing is very time consuming and has a lot of prep work as well as cleanup. Somehow, I'm always getting to bed after midnight these days, but I at least get my rebounding and Chi Flow in almost every night— that's my time and what I do for me to keep me healthy and going strong.

And as always, we are still believing for the miracle!

On the Road Again—Journal entry by DIANE HUSSEY—10/5/2011

Good news! Jerry is out on a sales trip and feeling really good! The weather is beautiful, sunny and warm, and just a great time to get out and make calls.

It felt a bit like Christmas last night as we made the list and checked it twice as to all that he needs to go on the trip:

Immersion blender, coffee grinder, cottage cheese, flaxseed, flaxseed oil, silverware, measuring spoons, bowl, plate, juice, honey, supplements, food for breakfasts, lunches, and dinners.

So all is well. Thank you all for your prayers. We continue to stand in faith that this will be how Jerry feels EVERY day—not because he had a blood transfusion a couple days ago, but because he is HEALED in Jesus' Name!

The Conundrum Leads to Semi-retirement—Journal entry by DIANE HUSSEY—10/12/2011

I love that word, conundrum, which means puzzle or mystery.

Jerry felt really good Sunday and was planning on taking a sales trip again this week. He felt good as he left for the doctor's office Monday morning, but his blood work was not very good—defying how he felt physically, and therein lies the conundrum.

How is it that he can feel so good and look good, and have numbers that look so bad? (I say, "That's what faith, hope, and a positive mental attitude look like!") *So instead of going out of town, he received a couple of bags of platelets Tuesday and two units of blood today.*

Jerry's employer has been super through this whole cancer ordeal, and we couldn't be more appreciative of their support, but it just isn't fair to them. They need someone who can work and cover the territory, so Jerry has decided to semi-retire. He loves his job and the folks at work, so he will continue to do what he can in training his replacement and going into the office or working from home. He has an incredible memory regarding his customers, their needs, orders, scheduling, and potential. Often he was a trouble shooter for the customer, as well as for his employer.

Today he applied for Social Security. Does that officially make him an "old fart"?

> *There is an incredibly fine line between having the faith that will move mountains and complete denial. I think we've been blessed to get a reality check so that we can fine-tune the prayers, while taking care of some of the more practical matters that have been set on the back burner for too long.*
>
> *Monday's report was one of those "gut punches" that knock the wind out of your sails. It's hard to keep your eyes on Jesus when you're bent over, but our eyes are back up and focused on the Great Healer, and still praying for the miracle.*
>
> *With Christ ALL things are possible!*

The following was not posted in CaringBridge, but I felt it important to share.

We have shared a lot about our faith, Jerry's and mine, and I have a very strong personal relationship with God. In 1 Kings 19:12, the Bible talks about God's "still, small voice," how he speaks within our thoughts and hearts in something like whispers. I am often blessed to receive words of knowledge, visions, and to hear His still, small voice. In my prayer closet (the bedroom walk-in closet), I've found a special connection with God. Our time with Him isn't all about praying. We also need to stop talking and learn to listen. I'm thankful that I finally learned to stop and listen so I can hear Him.

I kept the following interaction to myself, not wanting to acknowledge it publicly via CaringBridge because I didn't want Jerry or anyone else to think I was giving up, nor did I want them to give up.

I was in my prayer closet, praying for a miracle for Jerry, when God spoke, and I lovingly heard, "There's not going to be another miracle. He's already had two."

I understood His meaning. Jerry lived ten years after being diagnosed with lung cancer, which is usually five years maximum. He survived six years after his second lung cancer diagnosis, when he was given four to six months. I tried to process "no miracle," but didn't want to accept it.

It was during that same prayer time that God had to shock me to get my attention. This was about a week before my birthday, and I had an overwhelming sense that Jerry was going to die on my birthday. I felt like I was wrestling with God, trying to wrap my head around it, sobbing, and crying out for His help. I questioned Him—had I heard right?

I stopped, waited, and listened for that still, small voice again. "Full circle."

I'd been receiving the message "full circle" from God for some time—the Alpha and the Omega, the first and the last, the beginning and the end. Within minutes, I understood and found peace. My birth, Jerry's death—full circle. If that happened, God was in it, and I would be okay with it.

God had given me forewarning, and I was thankful He had.

I continued praying, and then God gave me a special gift, the prayer to pray for Jerry going forward. "Grace, mercy, and no pain." It is such a simple and yet positive prayer for someone who has a terminal illness. So that is what I regularly prayed, "Grace, mercy, and no pain." And our journey continued.

As before, I still encouraged faith in God's healing when I journaled at CaringBridge, partly because I knew that God had given my Jerry two health miracles, and that He blesses many with similar miracles, even when they don't realize it; because God hears and answers prayers; because He cares and loves. And partly because I wasn't fully ready to accept saying good-bye to Jerry.

Thankfully, Jerry didn't die on my birthday. God had a much better plan.

☐

2+2+2—Journal entry by DIANE HUSSEY—*10/19/2011*

We're getting an understanding of how it works now—2 units of blood and 2 units of platelets plus 2 shots = feeling pretty darn good!

So, blood and platelets every week. Side effects: very tired when he gets home from the Benadryl they give before the transfusion to minimize any allergic reactions, and heart palpitations the next day. After twenty-four hours though, Jerry feels pretty good.

So basically, Jerry feels good about half the time. By Sunday he's dragging, and by Wednesday afternoon he's back to feeling pretty fair.

Please pray for restoration of his veins, restoration of his body's ability to make red blood cells, and restoration of his immune system. When that happens, he will be cured, and he won't have to rely on 2+2+2.

Walking in faith!

TURNING THE CORNER!—Journal entry by DIANE HUSSEY—10/24/2011

Maybe that should be Turning the CornerS!

Last week Jerry filed for Social Security and his company had a semi-retirement party for him. They had such nice things to say about him—made me wonder how much he had to pay them to say all those nice things. :)

Seriously, it was a wonderful dinner and wonderful memories. Jerry had worked for the owner previously and has known him for thirty-eight years. Two of the other employees (out of a staff of thirteen) had also worked with Jerry previously, so there is a very long history with this group. My parents came out for the dinner, and my dad had also worked at that same company, so he knew them as well. (Shall we all start singing? "It's a Small World. . . .")

Of course, this morning it was off to work because Jerry is only SEMI-retired and loves what he does.

One of the reasons he decided to semi-retire is because of the doctor appointments and time getting transfusions. So today he went into the doctor and found that semi-retirement is really agreeing with him! His numbers were so good on the blood test that he doesn't need a blood transfusion this week!!!

So, prayers are being answered, and/or the alternative treatments are kicking in. I prefer to think God's hand is guiding the treatment—giving Him all the credit first and foremost.

Not only are we excited, but the doctor was ecstatic as well. So please keep praying—we've turned the corner and are on the road to recovery!!!!!!!!!!!!!!!

As always, STANDING IN FAITH AND BELIEVING FOR HEALING!

Ten days passed before I journaled again.

Riding the Roller Coaster—Journal entry by DIANE HUSSEY—11/3/2011

Sometimes it feels like we're turning corners and going down new roads. Other times it feels like a roller coaster—up and down.

This week has been a roller coaster. His energy level is down, and he didn't rebound like he usually does after a transfusion. Finding a vein to draw blood or to insert an IV has been especially challenging for the nurses and techs. They needed to draw blood three times—it took six tries. They needed to insert the IV—that also took six attempts. Jerry has been a veritable pincushion.

The good news is that he will be getting a port on Tuesday. We talked to the surgeon today, and everything has been coordinated—receiving blood and platelets, if needed, before the surgery.

We had been planning to go to North Carolina to visit family and friends during Thanksgiving, but given Jerry's present health condition, we've opted to stay home and have our kids come up instead. We would have loved to have been able to visit with so many who have been following Jerry's journey, but it probably would have been a very foolish attempt, given the time of year and his health. (We were snowbound in Ohio while returning from a trip to North Carolina for Thanksgiving thirty-seven years ago.)

We were feeling a real need to recharge our batteries mentally, yesterday and today, so we went out for a cheeseburger yesterday, and had pizza for lunch today. Jerry has been craving Buffalo Wild Wings, so we went out this evening for them. I think we've had our fill of junk food for a while, but it was good for us to get out together and splurge a bit.

I want everyone to know that I've made a HUGE sacrifice for Jerry. Because it is getting SO cold and windy, I'm giving him my garage, so he doesn't have to walk so far to his garage and doesn't have to get into a cold vehicle. It was one of the requirements when he was shopping for our home— a two-plus-car detached garage for him for his woodworking, and an attached garage for me for my car (especially for winters). So now I've given up my garage. Let me tell you, that is TRUE LOVE! :)

I'd just like to ask for prayers that Jerry is healthy enough to go through the surgery on Tuesday and for success in the installation of the port. They will be able to draw blood from it as well as give him IVs and transfusions. It will be below the skin, so it should make his life so much easier.

We're still cruising along in this journey called life, praying for all good things and seeing God's glory in the midst of the ride. We pray that you are enjoying your own ride and find the good in all the challenges.

Laughing All the Way!—Journal entry by DIANE HUSSEY—*11/8/2011*

Tara arrived Saturday evening and will be here for a while (we're not sure how long), but our family's answer to anything related to time is "two weeks," so we're just saying, "Two weeks." (If you don't know what "two weeks" is, rent the movie The Money Pit *with Tom Hanks and Shelley Long and laugh with us.) So, when we simply say, "Two weeks," it's likely to send Tara and me into uncontrolled laughter.*

And we're like a dog with a bone—when something tickles us, we don't let it go, and continue to build on the stories. Sometimes Jerry gets it, sometimes he doesn't, but he laughs at our silliness, and sometimes we have to explain it.

We don't try to be loud and disruptive. We laugh and it just happens. Today the nurses closed the door and office window at the doctor's office (maybe they were upset they couldn't be part of our fun). Maybe our laughter seems inappropriate to some given the severity of the usual doctor/hospital environment, but don't they say laughter is the best medicine?

Hopefully these little tidbits make you laugh with us. We have laughed so hard we can hardly breathe. And yes, we do have a very warped sense of humor sometimes.

We were always giggling and saying, "What's the plan? Do we have a plan? I need a PLAN!" (in reference to the surgeon who was supposed to install the port for the bone marrow treatment a few months earlier).

Tara, ever the efficient one and a medical technician, asked me on the trip home from the airport if we had all our papers in order, including a DNR. I told her everything but the DNR. She casually started the discussion about a DNR with Jerry this morning at breakfast.

He responded, "Do I need one?"

Tara: "It's up to you."

Jerry: "I don't know what DNR stands for—Department of Natural Resources so you can throw my ash over there?"

We were laughing hysterically, crying in laughter, as he still didn't know what DNR stood for.

It's even funnier when you understand the context of Jerry's wishes. He would like to be cremated and have his ashes spread at a specific national park.

Tara and I were laughing so hard we could hardly breathe. Jerry was laughing at us laughing. Are we warped or what? Oh, and for those who don't know what DNR stands for—it's Do Not Resuscitate, hardly a laughing matter most of the time.

Then we were waiting for his prescription at Walmart, and there was some confusion with the antibiotic that had been prescribed. The pharmacist (Anna) called the doctor and then came out to discuss the prescription. With Tara's medical knowledge, Jerry asked Tara what the decision was.

Tara's response: "Anna called the doctor, and the doctor said, 'No more monkeys jumping on the bed.' "

Jerry didn't get it—never sang the song with the kids.

She and I are laughing hysterically, trying to explain it, and poor Jerry is just mystified by us, trying to understand about monkeys, and jumping on the bed, and what does that have to do with his antibiotic?

We thought Tara had explained it to Jerry's understanding, but several hours later, at dinner, he again questioned the monkeys jumping on the bed when he asked, "Did the doctor really say no more jumping on the bed?"

Laughing is SO good for the body, mind, and soul!

Okay, here are the words.

Five little monkeys jumping on the bed,
One fell off and bumped his head.
Mama called the doctor, and the doctor said,
No more monkeys jumping on the bed.

Four little monkeys jumping on the bed . . .
down to . . .
No more monkeys jumping on the bed!

(This had absolutely nothing to do with the antibiotic, other than a doctor was in the lyrics. It was simply a tangent, an unrelated joke that left Tara and me laughing hysterically.)

Anything can set us off into laughter. Jerry came down after his nap with his new, nice and warm, fleece sweatpants on. We cracked up to see the stickers running down his leg—a definite Minnie Pearl look.

*We have a plan! We are getting ready to head to the hospital for platelets and port installation. None of us are planning on jumping on any beds. :) And we have all our **D**ucks i**N** a **R**ow. A New DNR!!!!*

I hope you have had a few laughs—it's good for what ails you!

Believing. . . .

(Below and in some of the following journal entries, I have included some comments that were posted to the CaringBridge website by family and friends. They appear in a different font to make them distinctive.)

11/8/2011—Keep on laughing and sharing the stories. I'm still singing the monkey song. Can't seem to get it out of my head since you shared the story. Love and prayers!

11/8/2011—Love your laughing stories. So glad Tara is home. Thinking and praying for you often.

11/8/2011—I wish I could be so positive and cheerful on a normal day.

11/8/2011—Okay, you guys, now you've got the tears rolling down my cheeks from laughter! Poor Jerry, he'll never understand the humor that we women can find in things, will he? That's what I think sometimes when he responds to our e-mail humor—he just doesn't get it, but the goal is to keep him laughing. Glad to have received the great news about his port. That man just keeps on keeping on! God loves you all, and by all means, keep up the laughter!

11/8/2011—Reading this post made me smile. It reminded me of so many situations I had with both my parents and siblings during what was supposed to be such a terrible time in our lives. We just laughed and laughed. We had the doctors and nurses at Loyola thinking we were all nuts! Laughing is good. Laughing makes you happy! I am so happy to see another family laughing together during uncertain times. Keep laughing!

The Report on the Port—Journal entry by DIANE HUSSEY—11/9/2011
Success! The port is in, and Jerry is home. Jerry was wondering on the way to the hospital if the port is installed on the right side, is it still called a port or is it a starboard? (For all non-sailors, port means left and starboard means right.) Yes, the humor continues.

Not only did they install a port, it's a power port! So, we're praying he gets power to spare!

Jerry was a real trooper through the whole thing. Prayers were answered—the nurse got the IV in on the first try, and it was painless. Now all blood draws and IVs will be easy! They gave him Benadryl during the platelet transfusion, so he faded in and out of consciousness most of the time and slept through all the fun.

Tara and I had lots of laughs. She pretended to be a camouflaged ninja warrior moving from one side of the room to the other. It was hysterical to see her trying to hide behind the hospital table and IV pole, and you could see her feet below the curtain. She squeaked to suppress the laughter. We posted it on Facebook, and truly wish you could watch it.

Everyone seemed to want to be part of the party going on in Jerry's room. We had fourteen different people come into the room, many pretending that they needed to do something, like look at his chart. I think our reputation is preceding us. :)

I'm happy to report that Jerry is resting comfortably—hasn't experienced much pain, sleeping a lot, and looking GOOD!

We just want to thank you all for all the prayers and support! We can feel them and see the results of prayers answered.

LIFE IS GOOD!!!!!!!!!!!!!!!!!!!!!!!!!! Celebrate life each and every day! Is your life a testimony, or are you moaning because of the test?

All praise and honor and glory to our Lord and Savior!

Always Look on the Bright Side of Life—Journal entry by* DIANE HUSSEY— *11/15/2011

*It's official! That's our plan. **Always look on the bright side of life.** Maybe LIFE should be capitalized!*

It was a challenging week last week, with Jerry feeling queasy sometimes, and feeling fine but vomiting for no apparent reason at other times. Strangely, it wasn't due to anything he'd eaten, because he hadn't eaten anything when he got sick.

Also, he's been incredibly tired, so we knew his blood work would probably look pretty sad. He received an antibiotic plus anti-nausea medicine at the doctor's office yesterday, then off to the hospital for two units of blood. It was a REALLY long day—got to the doctor's appointment at 10:30 a.m.

and got home at 10:30 p.m.

So, in spite of the challenges of the week, we choose to: ***Always look on the bright side of life!***

- *He did take us out in his 1965 Mustang on Sunday to eat, so that was fun.*
- *We've had some positively glorious weather!*
- *Our yard work is done for the winter.*
- *I still have roses blooming.*
- *Tara is here with us!*
- *Devin is coming up Thursday!*
- *Jerry went into work today!*

Tomorrow it's off to the doctor again to check the results of the transfusion and perhaps get some platelets. We are thankful for the port. It works quite well and is so much easier than getting stuck over and over.

The new picture is what Tara wrote on the information board in the hospital, under Today's Plan/Goals: "Always look on the bright side of life." It's a Monty Python song, a catchy little tune, but a tad bit warped—just like us!

Smile lots (and lean on God).

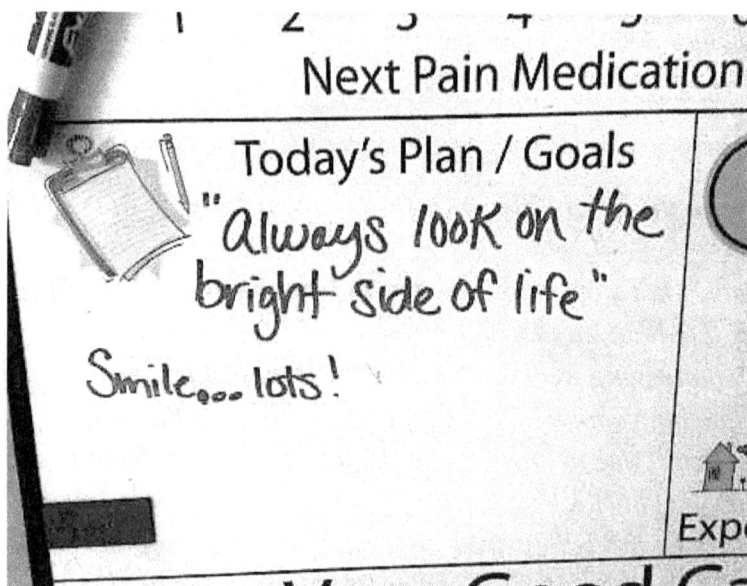

11/16/2011—Okay, Husseys, this is for all of you! I'm

whistling, laughing, smiling, dancing, singing, and grinning, and it's because of you ALL! You give so much courage and hope, and also the realization that you are right . . . as Jerry said the other night, "We're all gonna die!" However, no one is doing it with more grace than my buddy! Love you all! You know you stay in my thoughts and prayers, and now my prayers will be with a smile.

Hospital Entertainment—Journal entry by DIANE HUSSEY*—11/17/2011*

Jerry is back in the hospital. He started running a fever yesterday after they gave him another two units of blood, so they admitted him. His immune system is really low, and he has a throat infection that has given him laryngitis, so IVs of antibiotics make them think they can take better care of him in the hospital than at home.

Of course, hospitals mean you don't get any sleep and present lots of challenges. It's often hard to look on the bright side of life when you're in the hospital.

We seemed to overstay our welcome in the hospital this afternoon, and Jerry chased us out so he could rest. Devin came up and doesn't have warm enough clothes for our weather, so we stopped at a couple of thrift stores on our way home. While we were shopping, Jerry called to say that the port had started leaking, so we came home to let the dog out and grab a quick dinner, and then back up to the hospital with a few more things he needed or might need.

Several things had us becoming quite testy about the health care/staff comments and procedures, so of course that means diffusing the situation with humor.

This evening they moved Jerry to a different room, so when we went back up to the hospital after dinner, we found an EXTRA-LARGE commode right outside his room. We'd never seen anything quite like it, and it became a source of entertainment. It seems nobody knew where it came from, who it belonged to, or where it should go. We lost track of how many came to look at it, tilt it up looking for identification, and bring in new people to look. Check out the picture in the photo section.

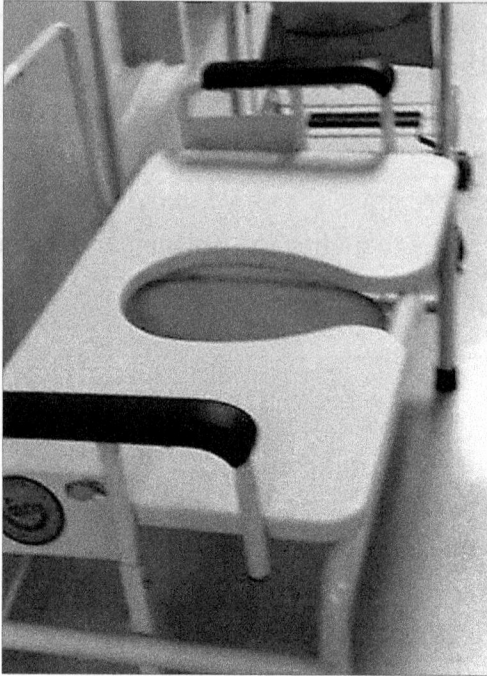

Tara kept us laughing taking pictures of herself making all kinds of weird faces, then texting them to Jerry, Devin, and me. We all had different text tones on our phones, and they'd beep, ring, or buzz. We picked up our phones and laughed until we cried.

Devin drew pictures on the information board—he's quite the artist. Then he drew hangman with spaces for letters. Tara guessed the phrase on the hangman game with zero letters guessed! Our family is SO predictable.

Then the tech came in to write her name and the name of the nurse on the board. I think they weren't happy that Devin was playing with the board. Of course, they probably should have introduced themselves when the shift changed. We managed to have fun in spite of the circumstances.

As for the important questions, we don't know how long he'll be in, or what the status of the port is. We'll update when we know more.

Our prayer requests are for a stronger immune system and the strength to bust outta there!

Leaning on and loving Him. . . .

11/18/2011—So sorry to hear you are back in the hospital, Jerry. We are praying for you. . . . You have to get well—you are too much a part of life not to.

11/18/2011—It is so wonderful to read how you all are

looking at and laughing at the little things in life. You all are wonderful and a great inspiration to us all.

11/18/2011—Wow, so you're leaking? Are you part of the Wikileaks bunch? That ought to "stir" you up a little!

More Blood—Journal entry by DIANE HUSSEY—11/19/2011

I was just getting ready to post my usual long discourse, and it disappeared. I'm tired and fell asleep and hit something on accident, so you get the very short version.

Jerry's still in the hospital, may come home tomorrow, had two units of platelets yesterday and two units of blood today. His white blood cell count is improving.

He was feeling much better when I left today—Wait, did that come out right? I hope you enjoy our bright and smiling faces on the newest photo taken Veterans Day at Applebee's. Thanks to Applebee's for taking care of our troops and veterans with a free meal! Tara and Jerry sure enjoyed theirs!

God's peace.

On November 20 we got home shortly after 7:00 p.m. Hospice delivered the oxygen and medications Jerry would need to remain comfortable. I was able to bring him home in the car, no ambulance needed. He had oxygen from the hospital and was able to walk into our home. He sat at our kitchen table with us, and the hospice nurse arrived to go over the medications.

Devin brought our dog, Connor, down to let him out. As you may recall, Connor was a rescue dog that had been so abused, he was afraid of everybody except Jerry and me. Normally Connor would stay as far away from strangers as he could and run past them as quickly as possible. He often hid under the kitchen table until it was "safe" to run upstairs or outside when the door was opened.

When Connor came in, instead of cowering or running past her, Connor went up to the hospice nurse and nuzzled her hand. That absolutely amazed all of us, and Jerry was comforted that Connor was going to be okay. Nothing could have given Jerry more peace than to know that his buddy was settled.

After the hospice nurse left, Devin and Tara helped Jerry up to our bedroom and into the recliner. We came back down into the kitchen and were talking when Jerry started yelling, "Hurry up! Hurry up! Hurry up!"

We all scrambled and ran into the bedroom, trying to figure out what to do. We grabbed a pan for him to throw up into, thinking that's what he was asking for, but he was hallucinating. They had given him morphine—not for pain, but to help him relax and breathe easier.

Tara called hospice to find out what to do. They told us to give him the medicine we were told to put in the refrigerator (that we were told he probably wouldn't need), and to give him another medicine at 1:00 a.m. And feel free to call if we had any other questions or concerns.

We were all a bit rattled and trying to cope the best way that we could. It was just a few days prior that we still had been hopeful and believing he was going to beat this. I could usually find peace in writing and posting on CaringBridge, so I started the post.

Home again Home again Jiggity Jog—Journal entry by DIANE HUSSEY— 11/21/2011

Well Jerry made it home this evening, and he is resting comfortably in a recliner in our bedroom. Devin and Tara had come home to rearrange the house to prepare for his return while he and I waited at the hospital for the oxygen for the trip home.

Our journey home has been made possible by hospice. Jerry needs oxygen and meds now to keep him comfortable. Our prayers for freedom from pain have been answered, as he really doesn't seem to have any.

At that point, I was interrupted. It was about 1:00 a.m. Tara had gone in to give Jerry his meds. She frantically called us into the bedroom. It appeared Jerry wasn't breathing. He was on oxygen, and between the mask and the noise, Tara couldn't detect a heartbeat or pulse. It was only because his head was tilted at just the right angle that we could see an ever-so-faint pulse in his neck. The three of us camped around the recliner, talking and praying. We decided that each of us should have some time alone with Jerry.

I remembered, from previous caregiver training, a hospice nurse who'd said that the patient won't pass away while you're engaging them. They will wait for the time when you close your eyes, lay your head down, or walk across the room to get something. I told the kids not to leave Jerry alone, and to make sure that we each were able to have our own time with him.

Tara asked, "Can I play a song?" and chose "Daddy's Hands." She held his hands tightly as she talked and sang to him and said her good-byes.

Devin chose "Cat's in the Cradle," and had his time with Dad.

Then it was my turn. Naturally, I wasn't ready to let him go. I talked and prayed and had to go (can I find a better way to say it?) to the bathroom. I told Jerry not to leave me, as I still had more to say.

I was praying in the bathroom that he hadn't left us yet, and as I was coming out of the bathroom. I heard, though no one was with me in the hallway, "He's faking it."

I'm thinking, *What?*

Then I heard it again, "He's faking it." (Remember, I do hear that still, small voice of God.)

Sure enough, as I turned the corner to go into the bedroom, I could see Jerry breathing from across the room and even see the pulse in his neck from the doorway. I yelled down to the kids, "He's faking it."

They said, "What?" and came scrambling up the stairs.

None of us could believe how easily he was breathing and how much better his color looked.

Often when people are near death, they have a rally day. He had a very short rally. It was intriguing, however, that he was hardly breathing when I left the room, heard "he's faking it," turned the corner, and he was breathing and resting easily.

Although I still don't understand why I heard "he's faking it," I think God showed up to give us respite to the difficult situation.

Our spirits were lifted, and we were given an opportunity to celebrate Jerry's life for an hour or so through some of his favorite songs. I know it doesn't make sense, but it's the truth. The mood lightened, we had some good laughs, and talked about music and favorite songs.

I went to Jerry's office to get a specific CD, looking for "The Wedding Song" or "We've Only Just Begun," both of which we'd used in our wedding. I really don't remember which song I was after, because when I saw "Alice's Restaurant," that was song we needed to hear.

There we were, about 2:00 a.m., listening to and singing "Alice's Restaurant" beside where he slept in his chair. We knew that in spirit, Jerry was smiling and laughing and having a great time. You see, our children had often introduced their friends to that song, and it had a special place in our hearts and minds.

That relieved a tremendous amount of stress, and we all felt like we should try to go to sleep. But first, I wanted to finish the post on CaringBridge.

I'm not sure I can adequately convey how much peace I got in writing the journal and sharing. I would pray and ask God for the words. Sometimes I fell asleep sitting in front of the computer, and when I'd wake, I'd just start typing. Often, I would think of those who were following the journey and felt like I was writing directly to one specific person or other.

When I walked into my office, the first two paragraphs were staring back at me. It was as if none of the chaos had occurred, and I continued after confirming that everything I'd written was all still true.

Home again Home again Jiggity Jog—Journal entry by DIANE HUSSEY— *11/21/2011*

Well Jerry made it home this evening, and he is resting comfortably in a recliner in our bedroom. Devin and Tara had come home to rearrange the house to prepare for his return while he and I waited at the hospital for the oxygen for the trip home.

Our journey home has been made possible by hospice. Jerry needs oxygen and meds now to keep him comfortable. Our prayers for freedom from pain have been answered, as he really doesn't seem to have any.

I added:

Our prayers now are freedom from nausea and from the side effects of some of these meds, as well as peace and comfort for Jerry.

We have kept a positive attitude and strong faith throughout this journey. We are able to continue that walk only through the strength and courage given to us by our Lord and Savior.

We pray that you enjoy your own walk in this journey called life and know the peace of a personal relationship with God.

We all went to sleep in the bedroom near Jerry. Tara and I were in the bed, and Devin curled up behind the recliner.

Tara woke up to let Connor out about 6:00 a.m. When they came back in, she saw Connor nuzzle Jerry's hand and lie down at his feet. Then he got up again, nuzzled Jerry's hand again, and lay down, as if saying, *Good-bye.*

When I woke up about 8:30, Jerry was still alive, resting comfortably and breathing easily. I knelt by the recliner. I couldn't pray or think. All I kept hearing in my head was this song running through it, "I'll Fly Away."[88]

I'll fly away, oh glory,
I'll fly away in the morning.
When I die, Hallelujah by and by,
I'll fly away.

I knew in my spirit that he passed away while I knelt by his side, but I couldn't bring myself to turn off the oxygen. I needed time to process, pray, and cope. I went downstairs and started making breakfast. Devin had gotten up and moved to a bed during the night, and he came in shortly after I'd started breakfast. Tara was still asleep.

About fifteen minutes later, Tara came down and told us, "I had a dream. Dad and I were eating snacks. He started talking about booking a flight. I told him, 'You don't have to, Dad, we'll stay here.' He said, 'I could push this plate out of the way and come give you a big hug.'"

That's when Tara woke up, walked over to him in his recliner, and said, "I'll give you a big hug." But he was no longer breathing, and there was no pulse.

When Tara told me her dream, we both knew Jerry had been talking about booking his flight to heaven.

He had told me good-bye through the song "I'll Fly Away." It would have been one of the songs he'd been raised in the church with, and the words were perfect for the occasion. He had told Tara good-bye through her dream.

Tara was upset with me that I hadn't told her that her father had passed away while I was kneeling there with him. She was upset that she'd had to make the determination.

Nobody gets everything right. But what if I had woken her and Devin? She never would have had that dream where her dad told her good-bye. I love that Jerry told both Tara and me good-bye. I wish our room had been bigger so that

Devin could have been in there with us at the time, as I'm sure he'd have heard from Jerry as well.

☐

Why did I feel compelled to share that part of the story? Because everyone deals with death differently. There is no right or wrong way. We were blessed that we were all of a like mind, that we could laugh and celebrate Jerry's life. Some may be offended, because they believe death should be somber and respectful, and I'm sure there will be other occasions where I will feel that way. But we must give grace and mercy to all to grieve in their own special ways.

Which brings me to the prayer that God had given me for Jerry five weeks prior, "Grace, mercy, and no pain." I had prayed it, and God had absolutely honored it. Thank You, Jesus!

As I've witnessed time and again, God is in the details. He has a plan, though we may have to step back to see it. Because He does have a plan, we can praise Him in the storm.

Now, back to the most recent CaringBridge post that I'd sent out to all following Jerry's journey. We received one reply that was particularly meaningful to me, on the same day Jerry passed away.

11/21/2011—Diane, please tell Jerry I love him, and you are all in my prayers. What I pray for is the same strength that you guys have had, and still have. You are truly a blessing for all of us.

Answering the Call—Journal entry by DIANE HUSSEY—11/22/2011
Jerry was called home early yesterday morning.

God answered our prayers for grace and mercy, and Jerry passed on peacefully, comfortably, and with dignity at home with Devin, Tara, and me by his side. We are thankful that he was able to go out on his own terms—at home with his family and dog. He will truly be missed.

We have always tried to keep our posts positive and uplifting. "If you don't have anything good to say, don't say anything at all." Today's post is short, with the essential information for now. I will close this blog one day soon with our thoughts and reflections on Jerry's eleven-year cancer battle.

We thank you for your thoughts and prayers during this journey.

Jerry served in the National Guard and Army Reserves. He loves our country and those who serve. In lieu of flowers, memorial donations can be diverted to the Intrepid Fallen Heroes Fund, http://www.fallenheroesfund.org/About-IFHF.aspx.

I pray we all will find "the peace of God which transcends ALL understanding," as found in Philippians 4:7.

All glory to God the Father, His Son, and the Holy Spirit.

(Over the years my faith has given me a comfort and peace that transcends all understanding. It's as if I don't go through the storms but rise above.

While that is wonderful, the process of writing our story has thrown me smack-dab into the middle of the storm, and I've been forced to go through it.

Yes, Jerry did die Monday morning, less than fourteen hours after we got home. We were married thirty-nine years, and he took a part of me when he went. But so much of him lives on, in and through me, as I share his/our story.

Nobody gets out of this world alive, and everyone's personal story and "movie" comes to an end. Though Jerry's physical life has ended, he continues to live on in the hearts and minds of all who knew and loved him. He will continue to live through this book, and all the lives who are touched and changed through his cancer journey.

For it is not about dying, but about how he chose to LIVE the final chapter of his life.)

11/22/2011—He gave a good fight. I am so proud of all of you for the faith you have in our precious Lord. I got a blessing every time I read your posts.

11/22/2011—Jerry was my "bestest" buddy in our school days, and I will treasure them forever. I am so glad I got to meet you and know you through our high school reunions. Thank you for sharing your Jerry with us and letting us know how he was doing. Please keep in touch with Jerry's "old" friends, and your "new" friends.

11/22/2011—His positive attitude and outlook set a

standard few of us could ever hope to match.

11/22/2011—Diane, Thank YOU so much for all the love you showed us all for keeping us updated on our sweet Jerry. I will always remember his ever-present smile and great outlook on life. In my heart and mind's eye, he will forever be that sweet little boy in my classes in Randleman. I know I (we) will see him again. My love to you and the kids. My love forever to my sweet Jerry.

11/23/2011—We met in Málaga, Spain. Every day since, I looked forward to your posts. This time I am saddened. My sincere condolences on the loss of Jerry. I knew Jerry as a warm and loving person always with a smile on his face, and that's the way I will always remember him. I wish you and your family love and strength. (One of our friends from the Netherlands.)

Chapter 20
Honor

Again, we were blessed. I continued to see God's hand in our journey. We were able to go to Thanksgiving and actually practice being with people before the funeral, which was helpful based on my funeral-day reaction to my cousin— she is *so* fake with her tone and sympathy that I told her to stop or I'd slap the . . . well, I'm not exactly sure what I told her. It wasn't that I'd slap the crap out of her (which was what I'd wanted to say, but I was able to say something a little more tactful than that). Then I told her we were celebrating Jerry's life, and if she couldn't do that, to shut up. (Again, not really, but that was the essence. God gets in my way when I want to tell someone off, and His words are always far more tactful!)

The Final Chapter—Journal entry by DIANE HUSSEY*—11/28/2011*

Today, we post the tribute to the life of Jerry Hussey. **You will find four posts, three to follow this one.** *At the funeral two days ago, Devin gave the eulogy, Tara read a poem and shared some special memories, and I shared my reflection on Jerry's journey. I pray you will grab something to drink, relax, and take something positive from Jerry's life and his death.*

In the pictures, we have posted the tribute that Tara put together—the cover picture of Jerry with the family portrait in the background. It was taken a couple of weeks before he was called by God.

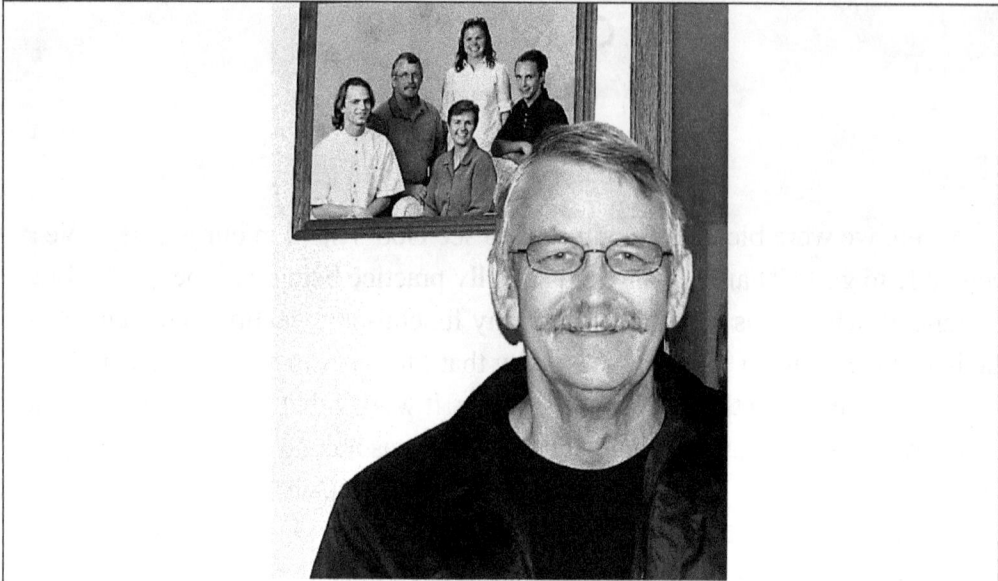

Devin read the quote from Kahlil Gibran. I read "Attitude," which was shared by our pastor just a few weeks before Jerry's passing. Jerry wasn't in church that day, but as the pastor read it, I thought of Jerry through it all.

"The Dash"[89] is a favorite—really something Jerry lived. He lived it because that is the person that he was. He was a wonderful man, who touched so many people. He was truly loved and admired. We are all better people for having known him.

Thank you to all who have shared our lives and our journey—family, friends, those who never met him, yet prayed, the CaringBridge guestbook signatures, cards, e-mails, and phone calls. You all made our journey brighter and easier.

To take a few lines from an Emily Matthews poem . . .

*There are some we meet in passing
and forget as soon as they go.
There are some we remember with pleasure
and feel honored and privileged to know.[90]*
(And Jerry was that kind of someone.)

---

[89] https://thedashpoem.com/
[90] This was printed on a birthday card I have from nearly forty years ago.

Tara's Words—Journal entry by TARA AND DIANE HUSSEY—*11/28/2011*

There are so many things I wanted to say about my dad at the service. I wanted to honor him through my memories and to convey what an amazing dad he was.

"My dad wasn't around often while I was growing up because he was out supporting the family. I am so thankful that he survived the first three cancers, and that I had the last ten years with him. As a child I remember us doing Indian Princesses together, sitting on his lap as he painted my fingernails, him eating nachos with jalapenos while cheering me on at my soccer games, completing our first woodworking project together for my mom, and all the projects for people in this room and others.

"I remember sitting in the garage together watching the rain and reading books quietly while just listening to the rain.

"I remember calling him or e-mailing him regardless of what state or country I was in, and saying, 'Hi, Dad, how do I . . .' and then we did so many projects from afar. Some of them included plumbing, drywall, cars, lawn mowers, and us working on our Mustangs together.

"I'm sad that I won't be able to ask him anymore, but thankfully I can ask him in my prayers."

Then I read this poem by David Harkins.

"[He] Is Gone"

You can shed tears that he is gone,
or you can smile because he lived.
You can close your eyes and pray that he will come back,
or you can open your eyes and see all that he has left.
Your heart can be empty because you can't see him,
or you can be full of the love that you shared.
You can turn your back on tomorrow and live yesterday,
or you can be happy for tomorrow because of yesterday.
You can remember him and only that he is gone,
or you can cherish his memory and let it live on.
You can cry and close your mind, be empty and turn your back,
or you can do what he would want: smile, open your eyes, love, and go on.

In hindsight, I wish I had shared more memories, but I realize I will still have my lifetime to remember and share them.

I would like to include one, though—one of my favorites. I was born on the Fourth of July, an Independence Day baby. My parents used to tell me that the fireworks were all for me. When I saw the movie Annie, I told my parents at age five, "I want my name in fireworks, like Annie's." They told me that it was something special that could only be done in movies. As my sixth birthday approached, I told them, "I want my name in fireworks." That time, I was told that they had forgotten, and I hadn't given them enough time to arrange it. Well, as all of you can imagine, I was heartbroken that my parents had lied to me—the fireworks were not all for me, and that it IS possible to put my name in fireworks.

Years later, I had some friends over July 3, and my parents sprang into action to give me a surprise seventeenth birthday party. My dad went into his workshop and hammered Texas-sized sparklers onto a board, spelling out my name. He asked my friends and me to come into the backyard, and he lit the sparklers. He had a huge smile on his face, while I had tears in my eyes, as we all watched my name light up like little fireworks.

Meanwhile, my mom had run to the store to get a birthday cake and had the brilliant idea to put seventeen sparklers on my cake instead of candles. It might not have a big a problem if she'd lit them outside, but as the sparklers sent a haze of smoke throughout the house, the smoke detectors started wailing. Initially, it was pretty to see seventeen sparklers on the cake, but they sent a layer of gray/black ash all over the white frosting, making it inedible. We all had a good laugh, and I finally got my childhood wish of seeing my name in fireworks.

Thank you to everyone for the love, support, and prayers throughout the many months and years.

Devin's Words—*Journal entry by* Diane Hussey—*11/28/2011*

"On Death"
For what is it to die but to stand naked in the wind
and to melt into the sun?
And what is it to cease breathing,
but to free the breath from its restless tides,
that it may rise and expand and seek God unencumbered?

Only when you drink from the river of silence
shall you indeed sing.
And when you have reached the mountaintop,
then you shall begin to climb.
And when the earth shall claim your limbs,
then shall you truly dance.
—Kahlil Gibran[91]

"*So now my dad dances, and dances well,*[92] *in heaven.*

"*Jerry Wayne Hussey was my father, but I called him Dad. My mom called him Babe. His in-laws called him Ol' What's His Name until they called him Jerry Wayne. His coworkers called him friend.*

"*He called himself a craftsman, but I call him an artist. Not just in his woodshop, but in his life as well.*

"*He was a great dad. He gave us the freedom to fall and get hurt, but he would pick us up, dust us off, and send us out again. I was four or five years old, and while sledding down the hill in our backyard, I careened off the edge and into a ravine. Mom and Dad had been watching from the picture window. Here comes Dad, barefoot in his bathrobe, in the snow, through the briars and brambles, to carry me back to the house.*

"*When I was nineteen or twenty, I crashed on a dirt bike, giving myself a pretty good concussion. As I pushed the wrecked motorcycle back into the shop, Dad laughed, slapped me on the back, and gave me a beer.*

"*Dad gave us the freedom to make our own choices, but he taught us that there are consequences to poor choices. As a kid, doing something that angered Dad was not a choice I wanted to make, but kids will be kids and push buttons and boundaries, and he was there to discipline and direct.*

"*I speak of Dad giving his children freedom, but he knew freedom is a God-given right. He believed in and protected the United States Constitution by educating others. He served his country in the National Guard and Army Reserve. He served on the Planning and Zoning Board in the Village of Prairie Grove. He served his fellowmen as an ambassador and senator in the Jaycees. He was a man of service: God, country, family, and friends.*

"*My dad taught me to work. For the longest time, I was certain the only*

---

[91] https://poets.org/poem/death
[92] Inside joke—Jerry was not a good dancer. The kids teased him at a wedding, and he refused to dance ever again.

> *reason my parents had children was for the free labor. I was roofing houses by the age of seven, with my three-year-old sister asleep on a bundle of shingles on a two-story house. The greatest gift my father ever gave me was his work ethic.*
>
> *" 'Work hard and pray.' He shared this gem of fatherly advice with me on multiple occasions, and I share it with you now because he was right. For a solid foundation toward a satisfying life, 'work hard and pray.'*
>
> *"It is hard to be a man in front of your dad. It's difficult to measure up to the man who taught you to be a man. I was blessed to have Jerry Wayne Hussey as my teacher to help me become the man that I am proud to be. I was blessed to have Jerry Wayne Hussey as my father. We are all blessed to have known my dad."*

Sometimes we must get to the end before we can truly appreciate the beginning. God had a plan for us that was far beyond anything we could have imagined or written. He wrote a script as only He can, and to fully appreciate how God shows up in the details, we need only look at how He brought everything full circle.

The original title of the book was *The Best Last Five Months: An Evolutionary Cancer Journey*. It gave me chills as I was writing and realized title of the June 21, 2011, CaringBridge post, "We Have a Plan!" was exactly five months from the date Jerry went to be with Jesus. We thought we had a plan, but He had it all along.

Jerry died Monday morning, before Thanksgiving. As we stood in Jerry's office, trying to think about funeral details, Devin asked what size sport coat Jerry wore. He had come up Thursday and hadn't brought any funeral clothes because Jerry had been doing well early in the week. I turned, grabbed a garment bag and said "Here, try this on." It fit perfectly. Devin gave his dad's eulogy in the tux jacket Jerry had worn the day of our wedding. Full circle.

Later that day when we went to the funeral home to make the arrangements, I was having trouble thinking and had to speak out loud to process. As we deliberated when to have it I said, "We can't do it before Thanksgiving. Thanksgiving Day is out. Friday, eh, let's give everyone the day to shop for Christmas. How about Saturday?" The family agreed, and that's how it was decided.

After we came home from spending Thanksgiving at my aunt's home with family, Tara and Devin went out to clean Jerry's garage. As they were finishing up for the evening, they found a box, high on a shelf, covered with sawdust and papers. They took it down, dusted it off, and brought it in the house. I had never seen it before. It was the most beautiful box that Jerry had ever made—a tribute to his ability as a craftsman, and obviously God-inspired years ago. And, as God would have it, just the right size to hold his ashes. God is in the details, and He brought this, too, full circle.

I mentioned that even before Jerry's first cancer I'd regularly donated blood and platelets. *But as you will learn later in the story, Jerry was going to need platelets, and a lot of them. Pay it forward when you are able, because you never know what you or a loved one might need in the future.* Jerry received 26 units of blood and 13 bags of platelets to keep him alive until Monday, November 21. You've heard how we decided to have his service on Saturday. Now you will understand how it all comes together full circle.

The moment of realization, about just how involved God was in our lives, occurred Friday, November 25, 2011, the day before Jerry's memorial service. I was about to head to the funeral home with the box Jerry had made when suddenly, I needed to know. What was the date we met?

We had met the day after Thanksgiving, 1971. But what was the *date?* When I looked up a calendar from that year, I understood. And I cried. It was exactly forty years, to the day.

We met—November 26, 1971.

Jerry's service—November 26, 2011.

Thank You, God!

And to commemorate our beginning and end at the memorial service, I wore the necklace Jerry had given me on our wedding day and the earrings he had given me on our last anniversary.

Diane's Thoughts and Reflections—Journal entry by DIANE HUSSEY— 11/28/2011

"November 26, 1971—Forty years ago today, I met Jerry. The very next day, on our first date, I fell in love with him. It is amazing how God has a plan for each of us—not chance, not fate, but God's plan. It is incredible, if we really pay attention to the details, how our lives play out, and often come full circle.

"Jerry started his sales career selling valves. He was from North Carolina and was transferred to Chicago.

"We met the night after Thanksgiving. I had gone to see a friend whose band was playing at St. George and the Dragon. A chance meeting, fate, or

God's plan?

"He traveled extensively at the time—gone for two weeks, home for a weekend, and gone again. He had a seven-state territory that did not include Wisconsin, Illinois, or Indiana. Four months after we got married, he changed jobs. Isn't it truly ironic how the man who hired Jerry out of the valve industry hired him back into that same industry over thirty years later? Full circle. (Thank you, Terry.)

"The Alpha and the Omega, the first and the last. the beginning and end. Forty years.

"God has a plan. He also gives us free will—the ability to make choices. Whether we choose to go our own way or to seek Him first and listen to Him will determine the course of our lives.

"I believed all along that God had a message that he wanted shared in Jerry's final journey. I hope I can convey the essence of our voyage.

"Jerry's journey home was public. Initially he chose to share it on CaringBridge but then asked and trusted me to write most of it. He talked and e-mailed and shared aspects of his life and beliefs. We have heard from so many people how Jerry's life over the past five months has inspired or changed them. It is an incredible testimony.

"We sought guidance from the Lord in this final cancer battle. Twice before, Jerry fought and "won" to fight another day. But this battle was different. In this battle he gave himself over to God. In his third bout with cancer, he'd sounded resigned as he said, 'If it's my time, it's my time. God's will be done.'

"But God wasn't ready for him yet. Jerry had work to do, God's work, because as the Bible says in James 2:17 (NCV), 'Faith by itself—that does nothing—is dead.'

"So, the first three of rounds in this fight, he had chemo, surgery, and radiation with all the pain and misery that is associated with that. His hair fell out, chills, nausea, and a LOT of pain. Let's just call that hell on earth.

"But this time we walked a different road. He put his life in God's hands and let God guide him. He didn't want regular chemo but was willing to try a stem cell transplant. When that wasn't possible, he embraced natural and alternative therapy.

"Sometimes people may say it was his only hope. No, our hope rested squarely in God's hands, and we prayed and asked for prayers. We believed in miracles with the faith that would move mountains.

"But we can't just wait around praying for a miracle, we act—whether by

our own impulses or reasoning, or by praying and asking for guidance from God. We prayed to Jesus, the Great Physician, to wrap His loving arms around Jerry, and for healing.

"But we also listened, taking great comfort from Psalm 46:10 (ESV), 'Be still, and know that I am God.' We put our faith and trust in Him and followed God's lead.

"Jerry believed that God led him to the Budwig Center in Málaga, Spain, and we were able to get one of the last openings before they closed for holiday. Our lives changed and revolved around the diet, supplements, detoxing, and therapies, fighting the cancer and building his immune system.

"The final battle was positive—the treatment choice and the change in his attitude spiritually. He lived, and I want to emphasize LIVED, the last five months of his life seeking a more intimate relationship with the Lord.

"I believe that Jerry embraced God's plan—the unfinished work. When Jerry found out he would not be eligible for the stem cell transplant, he changed 180 degrees in his diet, food preparation, taking supplements, and desire to be involved in his own health care. There is no way one individual can change so drastically without a transformation by our Lord and Savior.

"Jerry was a good man his whole life, and I have been so blessed to have been married to him for thirty-nine years. But truthfully, while the last ten months were difficult, they were also some of our best.

"The biggest difference between our first two cancer battles and this last one was that Jerry fought the first two battles, while in the last one he ran the race—God's course.

"As he reached the pearly gates, when asked to account for his life, he could quote 2 Timothy 4:7 (ESV), 'I have fought the good fight, I have finished the race, I have kept the faith.'

"And I'm sure he heard, 'Well done, good and faithful servant' " (Matthew 25:21 ESV).

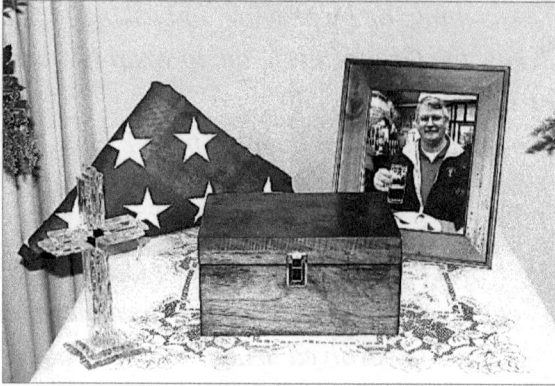

11/28/2011—(from his nephew) Very loving, kind, and respectful memories of Jerry. I wish I had known him better. I will always remember him taking the time to come and visit with me when I had a layover at O'Hare during my time in the Marine Corps. I also have fond memories of you guys coming down to visit on summer vacations. He was always so cool and fun to be around, not to mention a fairly athletic guy! I played a lot of baseball growing up, but I remember playing catch with him once. The more I brought the heat, he would do the same. (I think my hand stung for a few days.)

I've never told anyone this, but Jerry had a big impact on my career success, which has bestowed many blessings on me and my family. I always looked up to him and saw him as a dedicated, successful guy with an amazing work ethic. I wish I would have told him the impact he had on me despite the limited contact between us.

In all your comments, I see the many similarities between Jerry and my dad. A jack of all trades, and someone with an impeccable work ethic.

One more fond memory I will share about Jerry. I was about ten years old when Jerry came into town on a business trip. I would always try impressing him with some strength feat or athletic exploit when I saw him. Well, I remember him challenging me to stand on my head while leaning against the wall and do five upside-down push-ups. I recall being able to do about two or three before giving out. Jerry then promptly stood on his head and knocked out about ten reps without a lot of effort, as I recall! On one hand I was mad I couldn't do it, and on another, I thought that was one of the coolest things I had seen in my then-young life. And yes, about a year ago, while I was on a business trip, Jerry and I were messaging one another on Facebook, and I told him that story. Now I am so glad I did. I think he got a kick out of it. God bless, Johnny

11/28/2011—I can only say, I hope my son and family can say the same for me when my time comes to be with Jesus. What a wonderful testimony of Jerry from his son.

11/28/2011—That was a beautiful testimony to Jerry's life, and I truly believe he fought the battles and ultimately won the race. He was such a dear friend, and I will carry the memories of our friendship for the rest of my life. He did share his faith in God and that God would show him the way. He witnessed to his nightly e-mail "crew" on a regular basis and was a true inspiration to each of us.

11/28/2011—Jerry always found a moment during a get-together of any sort to say to me, "Thank you for your friendship."

Snippets from Jerry's Customers at Midwest Controls

Jerry's employer sent out notices to vendors, Jerry's customers, and previous employees of the company about his passing. I've included snippets from some of them. I thought it might help you know him better, to see him through the eyes of others. Each asterisk (*) denotes a new comment.

*My deepest condolences on the passing of Jerry. He was more than just an account rep. He, along with Diane, developed a great friendship with my wife and myself. We spent time together outside of work and I/we will miss that portion of our relationship terribly.

*Jerry lit up our offices when he walked through the door. With his southern voice and moustache smile, it was a pleasure to have him not only as a sales rep, but as a friend. Our love of NASCAR was always a topic of conversation. Jerry

was well versed in the products he sold and would do what he could to help the distributor find the items he needed at a competitive price. Jerry was a ray of sunshine and a brave man. We did not know he was also a hero. Jerry fought hard to battle his cancer, and upon his visit to us just weeks ago, he was still fighting. God bless you, Jerry. May you rest now in peace.

*I only knew Jerry for a short period of time, but he was always optimistic and a good guy. He helped train me in quality control and on how most of the parts worked when I started. He had a great sense of humor and knew a ton about engineering. He was always showing me how he was trying to test the valves and whether or not they had holes in them. He had several contraptions he was trying to build, and he was very inventive. He didn't have a bad word to say about anybody, and it was a pleasure to work with him.

*I worked with Jerry for a couple years, between 2006 to 2007, while I was working in the warehouse between finishing undergrad and starting med school. I can honestly say Jerry was a great guy. Although I was part time and the lowest man on the totem pole, he always treated me with the utmost respect. He always had a smile on his face. When everyone in the office was having a bad day, he was never pessimistic. I assume he dealt with his illness much the same way.

I wish I could thank him for being the great person he was. He always loved to brag about his family and daughter. I believe at the time she was overseas (Germany). He was extremely proud. I will miss him. The world lost a great person.

*I have always had the highest regard for him. He was the epitome of a refined gentleman and always treated everyone with the utmost respect. I know this is an enormous loss, but you may be comforted by knowing that he left the world better than he found it. My sincere condolences to you all.

*He will be missed on earth and, because of his faith, he will be loved in heaven.

*We have not done very much business with your company, but what we did was because of Jerry. My very first purchase caused me problems. Jerry went out of his way to make it right at a cost to his company and a great deal of his time. This is very rare in the present-day business world. His actions made me, in spite of the problems, want to give Jerry business. This means little now, with the exception it speaks volumes about Jerry's character and values.

*He was a good guy, and I always looked forward to his visits. We had some good chats over lunch, whether it be business, family, cars, sports, etc.

*We will miss his smile and friendly conversation.

*I followed his battles and progress via the CaringBridge page, and really felt he was going to beat that horrible disease. I was really surprised when he stopped in a month or so ago. He looked great and told me he would be back. I never doubted him. We had a great chat, mostly about cars, as I'm a fellow motorhead. I know there was more he wanted to get done on the Mustang, and I'm saddened he never got the chance.

*He was a great guy, and I always enjoyed his trip up to see me and talk about valves, mixed in with a little talk on the Cubs and the Bulls. We always had a good laugh, good talks, and he really enjoyed life. He will be sorely missed by myself and everyone he came in contact with.

I wrote the following CaringBridge post three months later, confident Jerry would want followers of our journey to consider this.

One Desire Unfulfilled—Journal entry by DIANE HUSSEY—2/27/2012

I'd like to preface this with an apology. I know this might be hard for some to receive three months after Jerry's passing, but I am <u>compelled</u> to write what is on my mind and heart today.

Yesterday I had some friends over, and we were discussing the baptism *that our church had a week ago. Reader's Digest version—I was baptized as a baby, and chose to be baptized as an adult, on August 3, 2003. My girlfriend had also chosen to be baptized as an adult, but her husband has not made the decision (yet).*

Suddenly. I remembered and blurted out that Jerry had wanted to be baptized. He asked the pastor about it less than a month before he went to be with the Lord. In talking to the pastor, Jerry had several concerns about getting baptized because of his health issues. (Baptists are baptized by immersion, and he was concerned about his fragile immune system and strength to get in and out of the baptismal.)

The pastor said that he would accommodate Jerry to the best of his ability, but assured Jerry that God knew his heart and mind. If baptism wasn't possible, Jerry would still be received in heaven, because he believed in Christ as his Lord and Savior.

Ultimately, Jerry was not able to attend church on the day he was to be baptized, and he wasn't able to have his desire fulfilled. Today it weighed upon me—did we ever write on CaringBridge about his wish to be baptized? I needed to know.

It has been an emotional roller coaster today as I have read the CaringBridge journal, with lots of tears and heartfelt memories.

I found that we hadn't written about his wish to be baptized, and I believe that he would want his unfulfilled desire to be shared.

*I think Jerry would challenge you to search your heart and mind—do you know where you're going? Do you have unfinished business to take care of? Remember, **tomorrow is not promised to anyone**.*

(Update—God has called me to His service, and I am signed up to take classes to become a chaplain. I pray that Jerry's life, our journey, and lessons learned will bring peace, comfort, joy, and strength to those in need.)

Committed to follow, and to God be the glory,
Diane

2/27/2012—He is in a better place with his forever smile.

Chapter 21
Spring 2019—Reflections

Sometimes it's the little things that mean the most, and I often share the blessing of bathtub crayons. A friend had suggested them for those times when you get a brilliant idea in the shower but have forgotten it by the time you've dried off and have paper and pen. Occasionally, I would get a download (faith-based insights) and fill the shower walls with thoughts and ideas.

While Jerry was on what would be his last sales trip, I wrote/drew, "I {heart shape} U!" When he got home, he wrote "I {heart shape} U 2!" intersecting at the "U." It's still there, on the shower wall, often bringing me a smile, peace, and touching my heart.

It's a tangible reminder of the love and spirit we shared in the journey. It seems it's always the little things—thoughts and gestures—that mean the most.

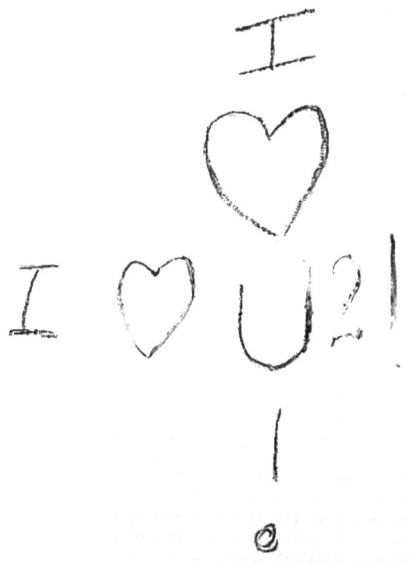

As I look back at our journey, I am at peace knowing that God was in control the whole time. That may seem to conflict with much of the tone in the book, when I lashed out at the doctors and the medical system.

While I was wrapping up my final edit, engaged in much prayer, Proverbs 16:3 (NIV) reminded me of my original intent. "Commit to the LORD whatever you do, and he will establish your plans." That helped me to refocus. Had I followed through with my purpose for writing? That there was, in fact, a better way to do cancer? Yes, but He had a much greater plan than I ever could have imagined, and He set me on the quest for truth.

Yes, God had orchestrated our lives for those forty years. He'd had a mission and purpose for us, though we didn't realize it at the time.

Crusade against Cancers is the continuation of that mission.

Jerry's cancer journey started nineteen years ago. We didn't know there were alternatives to chemotherapy, radiation, and surgery. We didn't know that side effects of some forms of chemo can cause other cancers.

If we had known then what I know now, we would have avoided conventional treatment completely, in favor of natural health options. We would have taken personal responsibility for researching and being involved in our own health care. Instead of chemo and radiation leading to a blood cancer, we'd have focused from the get-go on nutrition, detoxing, boosting his immune system, and killing cancer through natural means.

I can't begin to count how many times I believe the medical community failed us. Nor will I beat myself up or take on false guilt for something we didn't know. What I can do, however, is to share what I/we learned along the way, believing it was all part of God's plan to expose the truth.

In searching for the truth, my heart broke as I found myself grieving over unresolved issues. I wrestled with my anger that for years Jerry wouldn't listen to me about any of the natural health information I tried to share with him. Why was I so upset? In my mind, love and respect go together, and I felt that since Jerry wouldn't listen to me about natural health, and since he wouldn't take care of his health, he didn't respect or love me.

It was incredibly hard to write that, and it feels like my guts are being tied in a knot. But I needed to get it out. True confessions.

Some may feel convicted by what I'm about to say, but it's time for me to own it. Perhaps for you as well.

I don't speak ill of people, especially my husband, but his long-term attitudes about nature-based healing and his resulting actions, and inactions, are the crux of the emotional baggage that I've needed to dump. As I've shared my heartache with others about Jerry not taking care of himself and my resulting anger, many have agreed and stepped up to open a discussion with their loved ones.

Jerry made unhealthy choices, and it cost him his life. It cost me the love of my life and the life we'd planned together. I feel ripped off and cheated. I wish he were here to help me write, or that I were helping him write. I miss him on *so* many levels.

Unhealthy choices over the years take a toll on our bodies, and often create limitations and burdens on others. It robs us of quality time and adventures if we end up in a wheelchair or bedridden because we refuse to take personal responsibility for our health and selfishly over-indulge. (I don't mean to offend, so please forgive me if I sound harsh. There are many who are ill for reasons beyond their control and not a result of choices made.)

Our poor choices take a toll on our loved ones. Sometimes the journey is so long and arduous that it's hard to remember the person before their illness. It isn't uncommon for the caregiver to become so worn out that they develop health issues and pass away before the person they are caring for.

I'm not angry, and it makes me sad if I linger on it. Mostly, I look to share the lessons, in the hope that our journey will help others in some way. I pray that you are impacted to make changes, not only for yourselves, but also for the ones you love.

The reality is, knowing all that I know from reviewing Jerry's medical records, he really didn't have a chance.

I've learned a lot during the researching and writing process. To fully comprehend everything, I had to create timelines and spreadsheets from the medical records. I have binders and files of copious notes, medical definitions, research on chemotherapy, natural health, charts, and resources that document it all. While all that was a long, arduous process, dealing with unresolved grief was the most difficult.

Ultimately, I had to work through my emotions in my quest for truth.

Now, I'm at peace. God had a plan. He wrote the script. He had a beautiful ending orchestrated for us, and we were blessed. It has been a tremendously cathartic experience as I have found the truth in His plan.

Although I'm critical of many aspects of the medical system based on all that I have seen, read, and heard, we do need medical doctors and a health care system with incredible technology. They are essential for accidents and emergencies, helping to ease symptoms and maintain life. We all know people who would not be alive if not for life-sustaining medications, tests, treatments, and surgeries.

Thankfully, I believe things are starting to change and that more health alternatives are being implemented by individuals and accepted by the medical community. Medical doctors are moving toward becoming functional and integrative doctors—MDs plus naturopaths. These individuals realize that a proactive approach, resulting in better health and a stronger immune system, means less disease—thus helping their patients maintain health.

I do sympathize with oncologists, sometimes. Do they really have any clue how long someone might live? Maybe they do, based solely on chemo/radiation/surgery and all the statistics and research. If the prognosis is bleak, the cancer patient and their family may need to put their affairs in order and probably should be given a heads-up (like we should have been notified when Jerry's first cancer diagnosis was accompanied by hypercalcemia). But it can be a no-win situation. Some patients may receive a time frame as a death sentence and give up, while others take it as a challenge and determine to beat not only the time frame given but beat the cancer as well.

Sometimes the only thing that kept me going as I continued to sort through the medical records was that God was ever present throughout our journey. He knew what I would find in the documents. It was no surprise to Him. I believe He was the One to give me the messages that challenged me to continue searching.

Sifting. Contrast. Light/dark. Truth/lies. Good/evil.

In my mind, I had to get the message out, or my Jerry's life was in vain. My guts churned each time I concluded Jerry and I had been deceived or outright lied to. There were times I wasn't sure I could keep reading through the records or writing, but I would brace myself and take it to God in prayer. Eventually, I'd get a breakthrough and find the lessons that were meant to be shared—to awaken others through our life's trials.

We came to understand that the natural health approach was the very best way to face cancer and went from dealing with conventional treatment and its damaging side effects to experiencing holistic health.

We'd gone from being in the training gym with Rocky Balboa, getting the mess beaten out of us, to natural health, which in comparison felt like a walk in a meadow on a beautiful, sunny day with a calm breeze.

The contrast between holistic health and our experiences with conventional treatment were beyond what we had ever imagined possible.

Sifting. Contrast. Light/dark. Truth/lies. Good/evil.

I'd sifted. I'd weighed and contrasted. I'd found the light and dark, the truth and lies, the good and evil.

And now that you've read our story, will you accept the standard treatments of chemo, radiation, and surgery, or might you research and consider pursuing alternative therapies? Will you obtain copies of your medical records, starting on day one, and read them? And if you don't have a relationship with God, will you open your mind and heart to Him?

Part 3
Cancer Today

Chapter 22
With Sights Set Forward

Our conventional health care system is in shambles. We have doctors who are influenced by big pharma, standard medical protocol, and fear of malpractice lawsuits. Insurance companies and the government often dictate what will or will not be covered. In an effort to standardize care (in theory, to make health care better), patients may be labeled and sorted into boxes. The doctor can then just resort to what the standard medical protocol is—run some tests and write the prescription that matches the box you're in. There are doctors who are exceptions, but from what I see and hear, they seem to be the minority.

We have been indoctrinated, and our society has placed doctors on pedestals and heedlessly swallowed the overwhelming numbers of pharmaceutical advertisements on TV, radio, magazines, and the like. Many have resigned themselves to the lie that it is "normal" to have to take medications for the rest of their lives.

While there has been an improvement in health care from a natural and alternative health perspective, we have a long way to go. Thankfully, we see increasing numbers of people who are becoming open to new approaches. A lot of information is available now through the Internet, webinars, magazines, functional and integrative doctors, plus effective treatments such as massage, acupuncture, essential oils, CBD oil, medical marijuana, and many other alternative health modalities. Health clubs and fitness centers are springing up all over, as are organic and healthy food stores, and many people are taking responsibility for their own health.

Originally the manuscript was much more positive and upbeat, but that was before I started sifting through Jerry's medical records. I hoped our journey would be inspirational and challenge people to consider their options medically and spiritually. I prayed that it would bring hope and peace.

But when I came across those statements, written by Jerry's first oncologist to his referring doctor, I was infuriated and devastated. The oncologist never intended, I'm sure, for the quotes to appear in an evolutionary cancer book. As you have seen, they are exact quotes, and others are the words that Jerry's oncologists spoke directly to us.

"Marinated his body in chemotherapy."
"He survived it."

"Since I last poisoned him."
"A couple of small spots in Jerry's lung."
"He has a history of lung and prostate cancer."
"This isn't really chemo."
"I can publish that!"
"Psychedelic mushrooms."

Marinating the body in poison. I don't think the pharmaceutical companies and oncologists would want that in a commercial or advertising, do you?

The tone of the book changed as I did research to substantiate what I found in the medical records. The truth became heavy, and the book became a crusade, with a lot more science as I sought to investigate and bring clarity to the hell of our conventional cancer journey.

The truth of our medical system, and of cancer, needed to be exposed. The words of contrast—light/dark, truth/lies, good/evil—that plagued me before reviewing the medical records, had become reality.

As I searched for the truth in order to move forward, I had to follow trails backward to get clarity and understanding. I found that attacks on natural health therapies and holistic practitioners are not new.

It can be difficult to find the truth with a simple Internet search. Why? Because the Internet is flooded with articles of disinformation, trying to dissuade us from alternatives that work. History is filled with stories about jealousy and greed by big pharma and our huge medical system that relies on us being sick. In fact, we would be more accurate to call it our "sick care system."

But it is essential that we sift through the deception and illusion that has been perpetrated on us to find the truth. In fact, natural health versus big pharma looks like David versus Goliath.

A Few Key Goliaths

Did you know that John D. Rockefeller, oil magnate and founder of conventional medicine[93] (oil-based drugs and the schools that teach how to prescribe them), also founded the American Cancer Society?[94] The relationship between the American Cancer Society and big pharma—it's like the fox guarding the hen house.

---

[93] Insightful, though with clear political leaning: https://worldaffairs.blog/2015/10/20/how-rockefeller-founded-modern-medicine-and-killed-natural-cures/
[94] http://naturalsociety.com/john-d-rockefeller-founded-american-cancer-society-1913-never-meant-cure-cancer/

When I say there are many who don't want a cure for cancer, some people look at me like I'm crazy. Am I? If cancer were cured, how many companies and non-profits would be put out of business?

The American Cancer Society alone has assets exceeding one billion dollars, and annual revenue exceeding $700 million per year. The CEO makes over $800,000 per year. Just how much incentive do they have to cure cancer?

A Few Outstanding Davids

Check out the **John and Harry Hoxsey** story[95] for a better understanding of how chemo, radiation, and surgery came to be the primary methods of treating cancer.[96] No surprise here! Power and money crushed what had been effective treatment. Their story also reveals additional natural cancer approaches found to heal.

Discover the revolutionary figure **Dr. Royal Rife**, who used electronics and frequencies to treat illness and disease. Perhaps the following snippet will have you thirsting for more information.

In 1934, Dr Rife had a committee of doctors and pathologists oversee a study of terminal cancer patients. "After the 90 days of treatment, the committee concluded that 86.5 percent of the patients had been completely cured. The treatment was then adjusted, and the remaining 13.5 percent of the patients also responded within the next four weeks. The total recovery rate using Rife's technology was 100 percent."[97] And the results from this stellar work? His work and equipment were destroyed by the government.

Dr. Max Gerson was another brilliant physician whose work was met with resistance from the medical community. Doctor Gerson's work focused on diet, first to relieve his own migraines, and then to help other people with their illnesses.

When a patient reported his skin tuberculosis had been cured through diet, a clinical trial ensued: ". . . 446 of the 450 patients completely recovered, resulting in over a 99 percent recovery rate."[98]

The Pepper-Neely Congressional Subcommittee held hearings in 1946 to fund cancer treatment research. During this hearing Gerson was able to demonstrate a remarkable case history of cancer patients who had complete tumor regression/cure using his diet-based therapy after conventional treatments

[95] www.healingcancernaturally.com/medical-history.html
[96] https://thetruthaboutcancer.com/howard-hoxsey-natural-cancer-cures/
[97] www.wanttoknow.info/cancercuresroyalrife
[98] https://www.healthnutnews.com/dr-max-gerson-cure-cost-life/

had failed. What do I mean by "failed"? Many of the patients had been sent home to die after their doctors had told them that nothing more could be done.[99]

Gerson's radical idea about diet affecting health found limited reception by peer-reviewed journals.

The Stakes

If you choose to investigate the above gentlemen, you will find that the government has suppressed natural and alternative health modalities for more than seventy years. These men are just a few examples. There are *many* more.

Although there have been, and continue to be, quacks preying on the sick, there are numerous documented and proven natural health therapies available. I believe that years from now we will look back at chemo, radiation, and surgery as barbaric and quackery.

The stakes are getting higher. With the Internet, more information is available, and it is becoming harder for the government, big pharma, doctors, and the medical boards to suppress it.

Dr. Burzynski has moved to Mexico due to the persecution he has faced over the years. Others like him are paying a higher price to keep practicing in the U.S., though that information doesn't make it into mainstream media.

Natural and alternative health doctors are dying under suspicious circumstances. The deaths are often ruled accidental or suicide. But if you take the time to investigate, you'll be able to draw your own conclusions. If you Google "holistic doctors death series,"[100] you will read reports that dozens of holistic and alternative medicine practitioners have died since Jeffrey Bradstreet, the first, was found dead in a river with a gunshot wound to his chest on Father's Day of 2015. (The numbers keep rising. It's up to ninety, as of April 30, 2019.)

Other websites are trying to debunk this information and discredit it as conspiracy theory. I have done my own research and encourage you to do your due diligence as well. Who is trying to protect whom, and why? There is too much at stake in the cancer and medical industry to allow a few passionate naturopaths, holistic practitioners, and journalists to expose the façade of conventional cancer treatment, while bringing alternatives to light.

Rarely do we see the media exposing drug companies, because of all the dollars drug companies spend on advertising. Occasionally an article slips through, as shown with this particularly pointed headline from CBS News in

---

[99] https://www.healthnutnews.com/dr-max-gerson-cure-cost-life/
[100] https://www.healthnutnews.com/recap-on-my-unintended-series-the-holistic-doctor-deaths/

Australia: "Merck Created Hit List to Destroy, Neutralize, or Discredit Dissenting Doctors."[101]

We can only imagine whether the person(s) responsible for that headline and article are still employed by CBS.

The article titled "It's Official! Curing Patients Is Bad for Business"[102] is a scathing indictment of big pharma. It's a must-read. Here is a snippet: "Pharmaceutical companies are developing new drugs in only two therapeutic areas these days—cancer and rare diseases. Why? These are the only therapeutic areas where exorbitant pricing is tolerated by payers" (insurance companies). The article goes on to explain how and why we all suffer from this practice.

Are we going to sit back and let true potential cures from outside big pharma be crushed? Will we allow people and therapies to be destroyed or forced to relocate outside of the U.S.? Will we be forced to seek natural health treatment in Mexico, Spain, and other countries?

In setting our sights forward, we must look back to what was effective—natural health options—before medicine was corrupted by greed and power. We need to spread the word and stand strong to take back control of our health and our lives, rather than allow a behemoth of a system to dictate standard medical practices that are based on medical protocols influenced by big pharma.

This includes all facets of our health care. I've only scratched the surface.

Battle Plan: Chemo?

We must become proactive rather than reactive in recognizing not only the impact of big pharma, but also the impact of big agriculture, like Monsanto, and the effects of pesticides, herbicides, GMOs, and vaccinations, as well as the quality of our air and water on our environment and health.

Yes, it does appear that certain forces want to suppress natural health modalities, and those same forces seem to have no concern for the ramifications and repercussions of conventional treatment. Remember, Jerry was told to flush the toilet twice for days after his chemotherapy treatments because the waste was so toxic.

As I wrote our story, I kept thinking, *With hundreds of thousands of people going through chemotherapy every year and flushing the chemo, what is this doing to our water supply?* Then I remembered reading an article about all the

---

[101] https://www.cbsnews.com/news/merck-created-hit-list-to-destroy-neutralize-or-discredit-dissenting-doctors/
[102] https://www.medpagetoday.com/blogs/revolutionandrevelation/72407

pharmaceuticals found in Chicago drinking water.[103] I also wondered about the long-term effects of drinking minute traces of sex hormones, painkillers, and various other prescription meds. (Not funny, but a June 10, 2016, article revealed, "Salmon in Puget Sound would not pass a drug test," according to Debora Shore, a commissioner with the Metropolitan Water Reclamation District.[104])

Are there any studies on water quality and chemo? Absolutely. Following is a sample, and it's devastating.

The article "Environmental Impact of Cytotoxic Drugs That Pass through Patients" states that "septic systems and wastewater treatment plants cannot remove them" and that the "chemicals migrate intact into our lakes, rivers, and ponds."[105] (*Cytotoxic* means cell-killing chemotherapy drugs.)

Cape Cod, Massachusetts, is spotlighted in a study that examined external tumors on fish, liver tumors, and mutated red blood cells and DNA. Two ponds in that small area are listed among some of the worst in the U.S. or Canada, due to toxins from chemotherapy flushed down the toilets that end up in freshwater ponds.

It's chilling to read that article and start to comprehend the magnitude of the problem that lies before us. Here is a direct quote.

"Problem cytotoxic drugs are causing great alarm, both among environmental scientists and those who manage our wastewater treatment system. Service personnel who maintain septic systems know first-hand how much damage occurs when a chemotherapy patient flushes their chemo-containing bodily waste into their septic system. The drugs in the patients' waste are so toxic for septic systems that the septic systems collapse. When the system collapses because the cytotoxic drugs have killed the critical cleaning bacteria, all the waste, including the dangerous chemicals, passes into the surrounding soil and surface waters. If these surface waters supply local wells, the wells and the homes' drinking water can also become contaminated."[106]

And not surprisingly, cancers in such regions are fast on the rise. "Three-fourths of the towns on Cape Cod have breast cancer rates 15 percent higher than the rest of Massachusetts. Childhood cancer rates . . . 19 percent higher than expected."[107]

---

[103] https://www.chicagotribune.com/lifestyles/health/chi-water-testing-14-jul14-story.html
[104] http://chicagomonitor.com/2016/06/danger-of-pharmaceuticals-in-chicagos-water-supply/
[105] http://www.pharma-cycle.com/environdangers.html
[106] http://www.pharma-cycle.com/environdangers.html
[107] http://www.pharma-cycle.com/environdangers.html

Another scathing article, "Chemo Drugs Pose Serious Public Health Risks,"[108] is also a must-read. Jim Mullowney, an environmental chemist, worked with some of the vilest chemicals in the industry for nearly thirty years. When his mother was diagnosed with breast cancer, he researched the drugs prescribed for her. He found that the drugs directly attack DNA and pass through the patient. The chemicals are still active for two to three days and will be eliminated in urine, feces, vomit, saliva, and sweat. Anyone who touches those fluids, even the sweat, can absorb dangerous amounts of an active cytotoxic drug.

Cancer professionals handling the drugs at hospitals, clinics, and doctors' offices are trained and well aware of the hazards, but many of the caregivers are not and can absorb dangerous levels. What about family members, children, and grandchildren who live in the same home or visit while the cytotoxic chemotherapy is still toxic?

And we wonder why cancer is on the rise?

As a recognized expert in the field of hazardous waste, and the pioneer of the field of cytotoxic sanitary waste, Mr. Mullowney discovered that some pharmaceutical chemicals used in medical treatments are actually more dangerous than industrial chemicals used in factories. The disposal of industrial chemicals is highly regulated. The disposal of pharmaceutical drugs is not. We aren't allowed to dump paint thinner down the drain, but it's okay to flush chemotherapy waste down the toilet. Those wastes can eventually find their way into our drinking water.

I continue to learn, and I'm amazed at the number of topics I either never considered or gave little thought to. Jim Mullowney's organization Pharma-Cycle[109] has become one of my new go-to sources as I've come to understand the impact of cytotoxic drugs on the environment, as well on the safety of home caregivers and families. When I read the following quote at their website, I was chilled to my very core. "Once inside the caregiver's body, the cytotoxic drug will attack any fast-growing cell, causing cancer or other damage. If the caregiver is pregnant, their baby can develop birth defects, undetectable for years, or even die."[110]

I wondered, How many women have unknowingly put their unborn babies and small children at risk while taking care of someone who recently had chemotherapy?

---

[108] https://www.ecori.org/public-safety/2012/11/19/chemo-drugs-pose-serious-public-health-risks.html
[109] http://www.pharma-cycle.com
[110] https://www.pharma-cycle.com

The potential destructive impact of chemotherapy on our loved ones and environment is far beyond anything I had imagined. On top of that, those agencies entrusted to protect our health and environment from dangerous chemicals are either ignoring the conclusive research or choosing to kick the can down the road.

The following points are paraphrased from Jim Mullowney's TEDx Talk[111] and from the Rhode Island Senate Bill S0169 Hearing 4/11/15.[112]

- A study in the 1980s—before oncology teams became fully aware of their treatments' hazards—found that chemotherapy nurses had more than twice as many miscarriages, and their children had nearly five times the number of birth defects, as non-chemotherapy nurses (TEDx Talk).
- Of the more than two hundred drugs for cancer, twenty-seven can't be metabolized and are excreted in an active form (RI Senate Testimony).
- Ninety percent of those chemotherapy chemicals remain active for two to three days after treatment (TEDx Talk).
- A more recent study that tested the urine of cancer patients' family members found that family members had high levels of cytotoxins, even higher than the nurses in the 1980s (TEDx Talk).
- The twenty-seven chemotherapy drugs that remain active can't be cleaned out by wastewater treatment, drinking water purification technology, or any technology we have today (RI Senate Testimony).
- In Cape Cod, in one of the two ponds studied, sixty-two percent of the catfish had cancer. The government spent one billion dollars to clean the pond, but the fishes' cancer is ongoing due to the genotoxic (DNA-altering) substances that are still in the water (TEDx Talk).
- More than 98 percent of cyclophosphamide, a cornerstone of breast cancer treatment, passes through all wastewater treatment and drinking water purification (RI Senate Testimony).
- The most dangerous chemicals we've ever invented are actually drugs to cure horrible diseases such as cancer. It's irresponsible to think they have no effect on the environment because we call them medicines (TEDx Talk).
- "Any discharge of genotoxic waste into the environment could have disastrous ecological consequence," according to World Health Organization 2013 (TEDx Talk).

---

[111] https://www.youtube.com/watch?v=zX6OsvzZdOw&t=135s
[112] https://www.youtube.com/watch?v=Nq65Nh1WMj0&t=335s

- After a study of medicines and the environment—over three hundred pages and more than five hundred references—Dr. Christian Daughton, chief of environmental chemistry for the U.S. EPA 2014, concluded, "The best control measure for such highly toxic drugs may simply be the prevention of urine and feces from entering sewers" (TEDx Talk).
- In discovering that cyclophosphamide was being used to treat cancer, a researcher at a conference confessed, "That's one of the drugs I give my rats so they *get* cancer so I can figure out how to cure it" (TEDx Talk).
- It is insidious that our governments, our drug companies, our health agencies all know that this is a problem and are aware of the dangers of these cytotoxic chemotherapy drugs but choose to pretend that they do not have an effect on people (TEDx Talk).

Again, we aren't allowed to dump paint thinner down the drain—it's against the law. But it's okay to flush chemotherapy waste down the toilet, eventually finding its way into our drinking water and environment. Unbelievable.

During his TEDx Talk, Jim Mullowney shared that he'd met with the chief medical officer of the American Cancer Society to discuss the impact of chemotherapy on families and the environment. The officer had commented, "I never thought of that. We know cancer runs in families, husbands/wives, adopted children, but we don't know why."

Earlier in the book, when addressing how cancer seems to "run in the family," I quoted from the National Cancer Institute, that inherited mutations causing cancer only "play a role in about 5 to 10 percent of all cancers."[113] I'd assumed it meant inherited from our parents' lineage and our surroundings.

After all, in pondering the husband/wife and adopted children scenario, it appears to be an indictment of current environmental, societal, and job-related issues, as previously mentioned. However, the genotoxic impact of chemotherapy may, by damaging DNA, increase the probability that cancer *will*, in the future, run in the family, not only from environmental factors but also due to the increased genetic damage being done by chemotherapy . . . and by touching family members and friends going through chemotherapy treatment.

So, I'm wondering, are your eyes are opening, like mine did, to why cancer is on the rise and why we are losing the war on cancer?

Finally, the following may be some of the most difficult, but most important, information in the entire book.

---

[113] https://www.cancer.gov/about-cancer/causes-prevention/genetics

Dr. Theresa O'Keefe's testimony in the Rhode Island Senate hearing[114] is astounding and heartbreaking. She discusses two pediatric cancers, acute lymphocytic leukemia (ALL) and acute myeloid leukemia (AML). She states that *the number one cause of both is exposure to chemotherapy*.

I encourage you to watch the above video, but here are the facts.

- Both types of these pediatric cancers, ALL and AML, require two to three years of extreme chemotherapy for the young patients.
- One quarter of the ALL, and one-third of the AML, patients will need a bone marrow transplant.
- The minimum cost for a BMT is $800,000 without complications, and costs up to two to three million dollars with complications.
- Ten percent with ALL will die, while almost thirty percent with AML will die. *And the children contract it from exposure to chemotherapy.*

Dr. O'Keefe says, "That is what we are trying to prevent."

I am as well.

New Legislation

USP 800 took effect December 1, 2019. It sets standards for handling hazardous drugs, including chemotherapy, contained in bodily fluids. Thank you, Pharma-Cycle and all involved in your efforts, for educating and influencing those in positions to make these changes.

For more information and to find out the latest updates, please visit https://www.pharma-cycle.com.

Strategies and Scrutiny

So, we have information that has raised our consciousness. What now?

Now is the time to focus forward. Conventional solutions aren't the best for the human body, nor do they have the best outcomes for our environment. The same way pesticides and other non-organic farming poisons get into our groundwater, so do pharmaceutical drugs and chemo waste. Man-made remedies have their place, and even save lives, but if alternative, nature-based options have better healing outcomes without the damage to people or the environment, isn't it time we ramped up our self-education and took control of our own health choices?

---

[114] https://www.youtube.com/watch?v=Nq65Nh1WMj0&t=335s

Honestly, if you look at your family, friends, and society as a whole, are we healthier than we were twenty, or even ten, years ago? No. According to the World Health Organization, the United States doesn't even rank in the top *forty* nations in the world healthwise. Many Americans take meds to counteract the meds they are taking. Visitors to the United States cannot believe that we allow advertising for pharmaceutical companies on TV, telling us to go to our doctor to ask for _____ (fill in the blank with the new medicine of the month).

Why are we sicker than people in all those countries, when we spend so much money on medical care? Did you know, "Americans spend more on medicines than all the people of Japan, Germany, France, Italy, Spain, the United Kingdom, Australia, New Zealand, Canada, Mexico, Brazil, and Argentina—combined"?[115] Shouldn't we be healthier since we're told that we have the finest doctors, hospitals, and medical equipment in the world?

For all the money that has been thrown at cancer treatment and research since the war on cancer started in 1971, why are we nowhere close to a cure? Why have the odds of being diagnosed with cancer skyrocketed? Why do the American Cancer Society and the rest of the medical establishment no longer talk about a "cure," and instead refer to a five-year "survivability"? Why have they lowered the bar from hope for a cure . . . to hope for five years and one day?

If the medical community can continue to keep us fearful, and continue to keep cancer shrouded in mystery, they will continue to control our health and our lives. But if you pull aside the veil of secrecy and expose cancer and the medical system for what they really are, both lose their power.

Insuring the Approach

I have a friend, Kirk, who was diagnosed with cancer. The doctors, after determining that he had ample insurance, talked Kirk into a stem cell transplant.

Jerry had passed away before Kirk had gone through this procedure, or Jerry may not have opted to try for the stem cell transplant.

Although Kirk and his donor had been very well matched, he developed graft versus host disease (GVHD). The new, transplanted cells regarded Kirk's body as foreign, so the transplanted cells attacked Kirk and made him extremely sick.

---

[115] From the book *Our Daily Meds: How the Pharmaceutical Companies Transformed Themselves into Slick Marketing Machines and Hooked the Nation on Prescription Drugs*, First Edition, by Melody Petersen.

Kirk was essentially a medical prisoner because his health had become so precarious. He was in the hospital for five months.

I'd heard that Kirk's medical bills exceeded one million dollars, and when I questioned his sister, she laughed. "One. *One* of his bills was over a million dollars." And we all know that when you go into the hospital, you never get just one bill. There are many, many, bills—especially over a five-month period.

Important note: GVHD does not occur when people receive their own cells, and GVHD is less likely to occur, or symptoms can be milder, when the match is close. But the statistics are startling. The chance of getting GVHD is around 30 to 40 percent when the donor and recipient are related, and around 60 to 80 percent when the donor and recipient are not related.[116] Symptoms from graft versus host disease may be numerous and can range from mild to life threatening.

There are, I'm sure, many stem-cell transplants that do not have the severe consequences Kirk experienced. But I must be honest in sharing what I have learned. As I did my research, I often found articles with the hope and hype, but found the article "Bone Marrow Transplant"[117] by Mayo Clinic to be very honest and complete.

During a telephone call to the insurance company following Jerry's rejection from the stem cell treatment, a representative told me of a client she was helping through the insurance maze. The client's transplant had occurred over eighteen months prior, and he or she had been constantly in and out of the hospital for GVHD—for eighteen months.

In hindsight I can say I am thankful, and I believe God was watching over us, that Jerry was deemed ineligible for the BMT. As I ponder and pray, I can't even conceive of him spending six weeks in the hospital having his immune system destroyed, the potential for GVHD, and the limited life expectancy documented in Jerry's medical records, compared to three weeks in Spain and the subsequent months of beautiful experiences that we had.

I am sorry if it seems like I'm jaded against the medical community, but honestly this is just a portion of all I have waded through. There seems to be a familiar theme: "I'm sorry, there's nothing more we can do" is what people often hear as the insurance runs out.

The Elephant in the War Room

---

[116] https://www.medicinenet.com/graft_versus_host_disease_gvhd/article.htm#what_are_graft-versus-host_disease_symptoms_and_signs_what_are_the_types_of_gvhd

[117] https://www.mayoclinic.org/tests-procedures/bone-marrow-transplant/about/pac-20384854

So often the subject of death and dying will come up as I talk about our cancer battle. Death is the elephant in the room that nobody wants to discuss.

I believe it's important to at least broach the subject. In my chaplain's class, the fact was stated succinctly, "Ten out of ten will die." I like how my mom states it better, "Nobody gets out of this world alive." It often evokes a smile, putting a light spin on a typically heavy subject.

In conversation, when I say, "I don't think we, as a culture, do the whole death-and-dying thing very well," nearly everyone agrees.

I include the following small but powerful snippet from the movie *Patch Adams*, to challenge you to ponder your thoughts and emotions about death and dying.

(Patch Adams is a real medical doctor, social activist, and clown, who believes play should be part of healing—after all laughter is the best medicine. The movie is partly fact and partly fictional. Patch is played by Robin Williams. In the clip, Patch is addressing a medical board.)

"What's wrong with death, sir? What are we so mortally afraid of? Why can't we treat death with a certain amount of humanity and dignity and decency and—God forbid—maybe even humor? Death is not the enemy, gentlemen. If we're going to fight a disease, let's fight one of the most terrible diseases of all—indifference. . . . A doctor's mission should be not just to prevent death, but also to improve the quality of life. That's why [when] you treat a disease, you win, you lose. You treat a person, I guarantee you, you'll win."[118]

Because doctors are faced with so many constraints these days—time, medical protocols, dictates by the insurance companies or the government, and fear of malpractice lawsuits—I fear many have lost perspective of basic humanity.

Thankfully we now have hospice, so people are able to die. Years ago, it seemed like facilities didn't want patients to die (it made their numbers look bad), so patients, like my aunt, were bounced from the nursing home to the hospital and back.

Personally, I think we need to gain a healthy respect and understanding about life and death, for ourselves and loved ones, to be able to make better decisions.

And, in my opinion, when it comes to death and dying, it seems that the people who have a personal relationship with Jesus Christ, and know Him as their Savior, and believe that heaven exists, have a more peaceful journey. Those who don't may be more fearful, anxious, and even angry.

---

[118] https://www.youtube.com/watch?v=KDEjgOFOLho

God gives people many opportunities to come to Him. As 2 Peter 3:9 states, "The Lord is not slow in keeping his promise, as some understand slowness. Instead he is patient with you, not wanting anyone to perish, but everyone to come to repentance" (NIV). I think it bears repeating—He is patient, not wanting anyone to perish.

Many will argue that if God is loving, why would He allow someone to suffer major health issues like what cancer patients endure? There are no short answers, and volumes have been written to address it. If that question sparks something in you, I encourage you to start your own search for answers that bring you peace.

People often question God, yell at Him, or seek Him during the most difficult of times. They have come to the end of their ropes, to the end of themselves. They have no one to turn to. You may have heard the old saying, "There are no atheists in foxholes." When times are tough, when we're scared for our very lives, people will often turn to or challenge God. He is always there. He will never leave you nor forsake you. You may not get exactly what you pray for, but that doesn't mean He's not there and hasn't heard your prayers. It doesn't mean He hasn't answered, or isn't in the process of answering, in the way He knows is best.

God gives people many opportunities to come to Him. I'd like to share four brief examples that hopefully will bring perspective. They are super-simplified, offered with the intention of raising points to ponder and opening doors of discussion.

A friend was concerned about her brother. He had been sick for a long while, and she had been praying that he would embrace Christ as his Savior. She wasn't sure if he had accepted Christ before he died. I shared with her the story about Ian McCormack, hoping that it would bring her peace.

Ian has an incredible and inspiring story that I recommend when people wonder about the salvation of a loved one. He was an avid surfer and avowed atheist. He was stung by five box jellyfish, was declared dead in the emergency room, and awoke in the morgue. His story gives hope that even to the last moment Jesus will reach out to save you. I encourage you to watch the video online.[119] My friend, and many others I have recommended his story to, have found Ian's story extremely comforting.

Another example is my cousin's husband, who had a severe stroke and was in hospitals or nursing homes for more than four years. He was paralyzed and unable to do anything for himself. He wasn't a believer and was extremely

---

[119] https://www.youtube.com/watch?v=59mRZ1Vj8ZU

angry. When a chaplain, pastor, or priest would come in, he'd get extremely agitated, red in the face with veins popping out, and mouth, "Get out!" since he couldn't talk. As we'd hear the tragic stories of what he was enduring, my mother would ask, "Why doesn't the Good Lord take him?"

After pondering his condition for some time, I answered her, "I believe God is trying to get his attention, but he won't receive Christ. He is experiencing hell on earth healthwise while God continues to try to reach him."

Did God reach my friend's brother, and my cousin's husband, as He reached Ian McCormack? I hope and pray that He did, for "He is patient with you, not wanting anyone to perish, but everyone to come to repentance."

On the other end of the faith spectrum, let me share about two wonderful Christian men who experienced their own long health battles.

Andy was the most amazing Christian man I've ever known, who never had a cross word for anyone. Everyone who knew him throughout his life had the utmost respect for this small yet powerful man of God. In his later years (he lived to be ninety-seven), all who cared for him, whether in the hospital, rehab facility, or in his home, were blessed by his words and spirit as he shared his love for the Lord. Though he was frail and weak toward the end and had to be carried up and down the stairs, his attitude was always filled with the peace and love of Jesus.

Jim was a man of God and a patriot. His humble spirit and strength made him admired by all who knew him. I remember how he prayed for others . . . when they came to pray for him in hospice. Although losing weight and physical strength rapidly, he never lost his strength in the Lord. After Jim passed away, a friend asked me why God hadn't answered everyone's prayers and healed him. After pondering a bit, I replied that Jim had not only showed us how to live well, he showed us how to die well. He had been resolute in his trust in Jesus.

In my view, when we know and trust Christ as our Lord and Savior, there is no need for fear.

As I prayed about what to include about death and dying, God placed those four individuals on my heart.

Each of us knows people who have impacted us through their lives and deaths. Please take time to consider their circumstances and your own views of life and death. Perhaps it is important for you to open discussions with others regarding their wishes or yours.

And now to put it into perspective with Jerry's experience.

Jerry's cancer in 2005 was marked with a certain amount of resignation. At one point he stated, "If it's my time, it's my time. God's will be done." His words nearly crushed me. I couldn't handle the thought, or even discuss it. I buried it. I can't imagine how I would have coped if God had taken Jerry then. Without a close, personal relationship with God, I would have *really* struggled.

But God gave us six more years. Six years to mature in faith and understanding, each of us growing in different ways. Over the years, I continually developed a strong faith walk, while Jerry seemed to have a "come to Jesus" moment after the BMT was cancelled. It was as if a light switch had been turned on, and he was never the same.

If you've gone to church or Sunday school, you may have heard, "Jesus is the light." But I'm here to say, "Jesus *IS* the light!" And that Light brought Jerry and me peace, comfort, hope, and strength through the end.

I find particular peace in the following verse, especially when someone has been battling cancer or another challenging health issue. " 'Come to me, all you who are weary and burdened, and I will give you rest' " (Matthew 11:28 NIV).

Jerry and I both shared our faith through the CaringBridge blog and in person. We learned about and prepared advanced directives to let people know what our wishes were. (I highly recommend "5 Wishes," which appears at the end of the next chapter in the section Beating Cancer—My Top Twelve Challenges for You.) These should bring you comfort and hope as well.

I want to challenge you. If you could write your exit from this life, what would it look like? With all the medications, technology, and ability to prolong life, would you choose to be alive as long as possible, or as long as you could truly *live*? Just because life can be prolonged, should it? Those who know me hear me say, "I want to live until I die, and then go skidding into heaven." But in the meanwhile, I have a lot to do—live, love, and laugh!

God loves you. There is no need to fear death. Heaven is real.

Chapter 23
Cancer Treatment—What I Would Recommend

I have been asked what I would do if I were diagnosed with cancer, or the steps I would suggest to someone else facing that diagnosis. What follows are my personal opinions, based on Jerry's cancer diagnoses and treatments from September 2000 through November 2011.

I have done extensive research pertaining specifically to the cancers and treatments outlined in this book, and do not claim to be an expert on cancer. I credit God with the analogies that bring common-sense visuals and understanding.

Disclaimer

I am *NOT* a doctor or scientist, and I write from my personal education, extensive research, experience, and wisdom, wisdom acquired through the Bible and revelation from my Lord and Savior. None of the statements in this book has been evaluated by the FDA. This book does not claim, nor is it intended, to diagnose, treat, cure, or prevent any type of disease. The information provided is intended for your general knowledge only and is not a substitute for a physician's medical advice or treatment for any specific medical condition. Always seek the advice of your doctor or other qualified health care professional and institution with anything regarding a medical condition. Never disregard medical advice or delay in seeking it because of something you read in this book.

My goal in writing is that you move forward with more complete information, not dismiss or ignore any information.

So, what steps would I recommend, or take myself, if diagnosed with cancer?

First, it's important not to panic or make a hasty decision based on what the doctor or someone else says. After all, despite what we may think and the impression the doctor may give, it generally takes years of growth before cancer is detected.

Too often, I believe, decisions are made without sufficient knowledge. The person with cancer is often guilted or pressured into a decision by the medical community, family, or friends. They may never actually be able to express their wishes, because everyone else is telling them what to do.

Second, it is important to get a specific medical diagnosis as to what type of cancer it is. Whether someone chooses conventional treatment or holistic health therapies, or a combination of the two, it *is* necessary to know what kind of cancer he or she is dealing with.

Blood work is vital. CT and PET scans may be needed to show nodules, masses, tumors, or lesions. Is it localized, or has the cancer metastasized to another area of the body?

Also, don't be afraid to get a second opinion regarding diagnosis and/or suggested treatment!

Third, I would tell very few people about the diagnosis initially, and I would be selective in who I told. We all know positive people who will listen and support us, and others who are all doom and gloom and will drag us down. The phone calls, e-mails, and other correspondence, while meant to be supportive, can wear you out.

The cancer diagnosis itself can be draining. You need time to regroup and get your legs back under you. Well-intentioned people believe they have all the answers and want to tell you what to do (I was one of those people). While they may have a lot of good to offer, you can find yourself bombarded with dozens of different recommendations. It can become confusing and overwhelming.

When we do our research before telling others, we can then tell people what we have chosen to do with a positive attitude. We might say, "Thank you, I'll look into that," or "I've done my research."

Fourth, ask questions and *do your research*! If chemotherapy is recommended, ask what type(s) specifically, and then find out how it works and the side effects.

If surgery is proposed, what does that entail, and what can you expect following the initial surgery?

Please do yourself a favor and watch Dr. Peter Glidden's "10 Questions You Must Ask Your Doctor Before Starting Cancer Treatments!"[120] I need, however, to disclose that patients have been asked to leave the doctor's office for asking those ten, simple, yet pointed, questions.

---

[120] https://www.ihealthtube.com/video/10-questions-you-must-ask-your-doctor-starting-cancer-treatments

If searching for natural health options, my go-to source is CancerTutor.com. Money can dictate decisions, so know that there are countless low-cost natural health options available.

Investigate *all* options so you are able to make an informed decision.

Then do more research. Check the background of the doctors and other health care professionals you might work with, including reviews and references.

And do more research still: Check out my other challenges at the end of this chapter for links to start you on your own journey.

Regardless of whether choosing natural health or a conventional approach, it is critical to eat right and avoid foods and drinks that will decrease your chances of recovery. Especially avoid sugar, refined white flour, genetically modified foods (GMOs), fried and processed foods, and packaged diet foods.

Most people spend more time planning vacations than researching how to live healthy and avoid cancer. They spend more time planning weddings—and funerals—than exploring how to improve their health, and by extension, how to enhance the quality of their lives. You owe it to yourself to do your own due diligence.

Fifth, when meeting with your oncologist or health care professional, take notes or audio-record the conversation. Trust me, Jerry and I walked out of many doctor appointments thinking we knew what the doctor had said, but a day or two later, we'd ask each other, "What did he say?" A friend told me her doctor would not discuss anything while being recorded. Naturally I thought, *Why not?* From my perspective, patients need to understand and remember what their doctors say, particularly when the disease is one that can be life-threatening. In reality, doctors may avoid being recorded for fear of lawsuits.

Sixth, if possible, have a trusted family member or friend go with you to your doctor visits, preferably one who is calm and rational. Not only is it important to have positive and uplifting moral support, but the doctors seem to explain things better. You may designate them to be your advocate, and it would be wise to have a list of questions in advance.

Seventh, ask for your medical records so that you can 1) be proactive in your own treatment, and 2) keep the health care professionals honest and accurate. Often what Jerry and I told the doctors never made it into their notes. Other information was wrong. Do you honestly think that a doctor cares as much about your health as you and your loved ones do?

Eighth, we found the CaringBridge website to be incredibly helpful to us on our journey. It relieved us of making many phone calls, sending e-mails, and rehashing the same information over and over. The website is free, and when a journal entry was posted, everyone who had signed up would receive an e-mail notifying them of an update. We posted pictures and received hundreds of encouraging notes, prayers, and comments. Our goal, to be positive, helped us weather the storms, and we often found peace in writing to our family and friends.

Also, it has been very comforting to me to have that website to visit occasionally, to remember some of our very best times at the end of our journey together.

Beating Cancer—My Top Twelve Challenges for You

1. ***Burzynski: Cancer Is Serious Business***—The video that changed Jerry's opinion of the medical industry and natural health. The testimony in the first three and a half minutes is compelling, and life changing. Dr. Stanislaw Burzynski cured cancer yet has been persecuted by our government and eventually run out of the country. Less than two hours, you will find the education invaluable.
   ☞ https://www.youtube.com/watch?v=rBUGVkmmwbk

2. **CancerTutor.com**—This website is a wealth of information and the first source I recommend for researching. It lists more than eighty types of cancer, with information and recommendations for natural health protocols for each. It will guide you through the process and the basics of understanding cancer: the causes, prevention, chemotherapy, numerous protocols and therapies, clinics, and media resources.
   ☞ https://www.cancertutor.com/

3. **The Truth About Cancer**—This website is also a wealth of information, from articles exposing multitudes of problems that impact our health, to helpful solutions we can implement to improve our well-being.
   ☞ https://thetruthaboutcancer.com/

4. **Budwig Center**—The holistic cancer center we went to in Spain. A *must*-visit resource for anyone considering the Budwig Diet and a treasure trove of information on a whole-body approach to fighting cancer and other conditions.
   ☞ https://budwigcenter.com

5. **Dr. Peter Glidden**—Outspoken naturopath who tells it like it is. Watch his eight-minute video, *10 Questions To Ask Before Starting Cancer Treatments!*
   ☞ https://www.ihealthtube.com/video/10-questions-ask-starting-cancer-treatments

6. **Chemo and Our Water Supply**—Shocking information that few have considered regarding the long-term effects of chemo on our environment and the resulting impact on our health.
    a. Read the article "Chemo Drugs Pose Serious Public Health Risks."
    ☞ https://www.ecori.org/public-safety/2012/11/19/chemo-drugs-pose-serious-public-health-risks.html
    b. Read the article "Environmental Impact of Cytotoxic Drugs That Pass through Patients."
    ☞ http://www.pharma-cycle.com/environdangers.html
    c. Visit the Pharma-Cycle website for valuable insight in protecting patients, families, and the environment.
    ☞ https://www.pharma-cycle.com

7. **Chemocare**—In-depth information on chemotherapy, how it works, side effects, precautions, self-care tips, and more.
    ☞ http://chemocare.com/

8. **Health Nut News**—Cutting edge news on health, the environment, related politics, products, and more.
    ☞ https://www.healthnutnews.com

9. **Research Historic Holistic Figures**—Much has been written to try to discredit these geniuses. Learn how natural health remedies have been subverted, and you be the judge.
    a. John and Harry Hoxsey
    ☞ https://www.canceractive.com/article/Hoxsey---the-quack-who-cured-cancer
    ☞ https://thetruthaboutcancer.com/howard-hoxsey-natural-cancer-cures/
    b. Dr. Royal Rife
    ☞ https://thetruthaboutcancer.com/royal-rife-bob-beck/
    ☞ https://behiveofhealing.com/forgotten-genius-royal-raymond-rife/
    c. Dr. Max Gerson
    ☞ https://www.healthnutnews.com/tag/dr-max-gerson/

10. **Five Wishes**—Visit this website for advance care planning to document your desires for care and comfort.
    ☞ https://fivewishes.org/

11. **"Alice's Restaurant"**—Enjoy the song at YouTube, just for fun! ☐
    ☞ https://www.youtube.com/watch?v=m57gzA2JCcM

12. *The Money Pit*—Watch this fun movie starring Tom Hanks and Shelley Long. Remember our family's favorite movie joke, "two weeks"? Always leave them laughing. After all, laughter is the best medicine. ☐

And remember . . .

☞ Choose life.
☞ Choose your attitude (and make it a good one)!
☞ Choose to be equipped.
☞ Choose God.

I pray God blesses you with much laughter, vibrant health, new memories to cherish, and His amazing, immeasurable love.

Chapter 24
One Final Note to Share with You

Many months into the writing process, I started telling close friends, "I could write a book about writing the book." It took several more months before I realized that was the only way the story could be told.

It was as if everything I'd discovered over the past two years, plus the original manuscript, were pieces of the most difficult jigsaw puzzle I'd ever tried to put together. The original title, *The Best Last 5 Months—An Evolutionary Cancer Journey*, no longer fit, so it was like trying to put the puzzle together without knowing what the picture was supposed to look like.

And then, suddenly, the title came to me—a genuine gift from God. I certainly had prayed often enough about it. *Crusade against Cancers—The Quest for Truth.* I finally envisioned the "puzzle picture," so I could put it together.

Not long after, I was struggling with how to end this book and took my laptop into my prayer closet where God often speaks to me. I started praying and dictating my thoughts about the book's possible endings into Google Docs. Strangely, none of the words I was speaking appeared. Instead, I saw a random assortment of words that made absolutely no sense whatsoever.

Tired, I prayed and then lay down to take a nap. (I have a pillow and blanket in my closet and have an amazing ability to fall asleep and wake refreshed, often with a word from the Lord.)

Here is what I prayed before I fell asleep: "Heavenly Father, I come before You and ask You, Lord God, how would *You* finish this book? You have been with us since the beginning."

When I awoke, I heard the Holy Spirit speaking to me, and I turned my laptop on.

As the words flowed into my heart and mind, I spoke it phrase by phrase after Him (and the words appeared perfectly, as spoken): "This is a story of a man who knew of Me, but did not know Me as his Lord and Savior in a personal and intimate way. Jerry had to learn who I was and how much I love him.

"He needed to walk with Me and to share his journey publicly. It's not about 'if it's my time, it's my time,' or 'God's will be done.' I would have none of the resignation or giving up.

"He found the true measure of My love. He learned to lean on Me, to cry out to Me, to hold fast to Me. He was a shining example of how one person can live his life to honor and glorify Me.

"I want you to come to Me. I want this story, I want Jerry's story, to inspire hope and the peace which transcends all understanding. Come to Me, all you who are weak and weary, and I will give you rest."

I cried as I read it, knowing that it was the truth. God had been with us every step of the way. He'd orchestrated it all, so that the reality of cancer and of alternative healing options would be told.

I still cry as I read it, reflecting on our journey, and I've needed to share what we learned. It would have been far easier to just throw in the towel and never endure the heartache and challenges.

But Jerry would have reminded me of Edmund Burke's quote, "The only thing necessary for the triumph of evil is for good men to do nothing."

So that's how I'll wrap up the book.

"Crusade against cancers" are not empty words to gin up emotion and raise money to throw at cancer through a failed medical system. This crusade arises from my own quest for truth. It is my hope and prayer that Jerry's cancer journey and this book will send you on your own quest for truth, and that you will never fear the word *cancer* again.

It is my dream that we will each start a meaningful crusade against cancers, through prevention and natural and alternative health therapies, with God parting the way ahead.

I invite you to join the crusade.[121]

---

[121] www.dianebishophussey.com

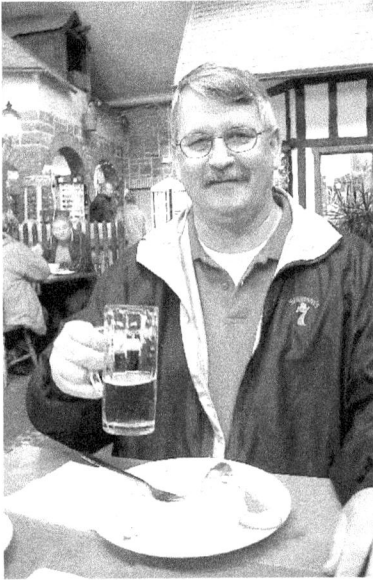

"If my experiences dealing with cancer
over the last eleven years
can cause only one person
to consider alternative, non-invasive medicine,
then maybe my journey has been worth it."

Jerry Hussey—CaringBridge quote July 21, 2011

Acknowledgements

Over the course of the three years it took to bring the manuscript to fruition, I've had love and support from so many I can't possibly name them all. But I'll attempt to, by dividing them into three categories.

First, those who encouraged me/us to write the book—who planted the seed—as well as all those along the way who heard about it and sincerely wanted to know where and when they could buy it. Often these were complete strangers who had a family member or friend they felt needed it.

Second, those who stood by me, offering mental, emotional, and spiritual support through the difficult times when I was tempted to throw in the towel.

Third, those who challenged me, and I mean this lovingly. I rise to a challenge, taking negatives and turning them into positives. There were those who doubted this book would ever get to the point of publication. (My parents, in their late eighties and early nineties, would often joke, "If we live long enough to see it.") I would see and hear the skepticism in others. I took that doubt and used it as fuel to continue, so to all the doubters, a big thank you.

Of course, I'm blessed to have some *very* special people in my life who deserve individual recognition for their contributions and help.

Yes, Mom and Dad, Ramona and Ralph ("Ralph Dear") Bishop, it *IS* finished. Thank you for your love, encouragement, and good humor to help make this book a reality.

Heather Moscinski, thank you for the introduction to your friend, the editor, (Tammy Barley). I will forever be indebted to you for that introduction.

Tammy Barley, my amazing editor who has become one of my dearest friends, what a godsend you have been to me! When we met, neither of us had any idea this journey was going to be so complicated and challenging. Thank you for your insight, patience, skill, and endearing friendship.

Dr. Lawrence Huntley, thank you for your friendship and belief in my ability to write. You've been such a blessing as you challenged me on so many levels. Iron sharpens iron.

Nancy Woerz Hill, thank you for reconnecting and sharing your husband's cancer journey. Your friendship and honesty about his/your recent battle rekindled memories that needed to be included.

Wendy Bouchard, Tammy Britt, Kathy Stevens, Angela Larson, Jane Andreas, McKenna Montgomery, Michelle Yoder, Olivia Michael, Stacy Curtis, Tina Wilson, Domenica Leschuk, and the Revive Project team, thank you, my dear friends. Without your prayers, love, and support I could never have endured the journey.

Lawrence DeSantis, founder of New Eden School of Natural Health & Herbal Studies, thank you for not only inspiring me to learn about natural health options but also challenging and equipping me to go deeper.

Jim Mullowney of Pharma-Care, thank you for your research that enraged, motivated, and inspired me to continue the crusade when my will to fight had started to fade.

Lloyd, Kathy, and Robin Jenkins at the Budwig Center, thank you for your continuing concern, care, and information for those seeking alternative cancer therapies, as well as your encouragement in the completion of this book.

Reece Montgomery, thank you for your inspiration and creativity.

Jared Silver of Executive Portrait Specialists, thank you for making the photography session enjoyable and giving me so many wonderful choices.

Jim Saurbaugh of JS Graphic Design, thank you for your knowledgeable assistance with the book cover.

Sheila Good, your energy and enthusiasm have been inspirational, and I thank God for bringing us together.

Jerry Hussey, love of my life, thank you for forty years. Oh, how I wish you were still with me! We had a great run, and I thank God for you and our life together. We certainly were blessed, and as I reminisce, I think of the Whitney Houston song, "(And) I Will Always Love You."

Finally, saving the best until last. Thank You, God. We couldn't have written it without You. Your plan and purpose took Jerry and me full circle— forty years. I pray that many are blessed by our journey and this book. All honor and glory to You.

References, in Order of Appearance

All of the following information was accessible when I conducted my research. Due to ever-changing websites and content, some webpages or exact quotes may no longer be found. However, if you apply similar search terms online (see s.v. "__," below), you should find comparable information.

Chapter 3

Footnote   Source

2	NIH (National Institutes of Health), National Cancer Institute, *NCI Dictionary of Cancer Terms*, s.v. "spiculated mass," https://www.cancer.gov/publications/dictionaries/cancer-terms?cdrid=44505 (accessed 2017).
3	Cleveland Clinic Center for Continuing Education, *Hematology, Oncology, and Pulmonary Nodules*, s.v. "cancer radiographic edge characteristics," http://www.clevelandclinicmeded.com/medicalpubs/diseasemanagement/hematology-oncology/pulmonary-nodules/ (accessed 2017).
5	Cancer Treatment Centers of America, *Computed tomography (CT) scan*, s.v. "what is a CT scan," https://www.cancercenter.com/treatments/pet-scan/ (accessed 2017).
6	Medical News Today, *What is a PET scan, and are there risks?*, s.v. "what is a PET scan and are there risks," https://www.medicalnewstoday.com/articles/154877.php (accessed June 23, 2017).
7	Mayo Clinic, *Hypercalcemia*, s.v. "what is hypercalcemia," https://www.mayoclinic.org/diseases-conditions/hypercalcemia/symptoms-causes/syc-20355523 (accessed 2017).
8	Mayo Clinic, *Hypercalcemia*, s.v. "what can increase risk of hypercalcemia," https://www.mayoclinic.org/diseases-conditions/hypercalcemia/symptoms-causes/syc-20355523 (accessed 2017).
9	Cancer Connect, *Overview of Hypercalcemia*, s.v. "what is hypercalcemia," http://news.cancerconnect.com/types-of-cancer/bone-cancer/hypercalcemia/ (accessed 2017).

10	WebMD, *Questions & Answers A-Z*, s.v. "what are the causes of hypercalcemia," https://answers.webmd.com/answers/1178124/what-are-the-causes-of-hypercalcemia (accessed 2017).
11	MedicineNet, *Hypercalcemia (Elevated Calcium Levels)*, s.v. "hypercalcemia survival rate," https://www.medicinenet.com/hypercalcemia/article.htm (accessed 2017).
12	NCBI (National Center for Biotechnology Information), US National Library of Medicine, National Institute of Health, *1,25-dihydroxyvitamin D and PTHrP mediated malignant hypercalcemia in a seminoma*, s.v. "testicular cancer and hypercalcemia," https://www.ncbi.nlm.nih.gov/pmc/articles/PMC3991903/ (accessed 2017).

Chapter 6

13	Answers™, *What are matted lymph nodes?*, s.v. "what are matted lymph nodes," http://www.answers.com/Q/What_are_matted_lymph_nodes (accessed 2017).
14	Science Direct, *Standardized Uptake Value, Biological Target Volume*, s.v. "what is standardized uptake value," https://www.sciencedirect.com/topics/medicine-and-dentistry/standardized-uptake-value (accessed 2017).

Chapter 7

15	AHCC Research Association, *What is AHCC?*, s.v. "what is AHCC immune supplement," https://www.ahccresearch.org/ (accessed 2018).

Chapter 9

16	DeSantis, Lawrence, New Eden School of Natural Health & Herbal Studies, s.v. "New Eden School of Natural Health & Herbal Studies," https://www.newedenschoolofnaturalhealth.org.
17	YouTube (video), Magda Havas (posted October 20, 2010), *Microwave radiation dangers in your home*, s.v. "Microwave radiation dangers in your home Magda Havas video," https://www.youtube.com/watch?v=aAnrmJ3un1g (accessed 2017).

18	The Truth About Cancer®, *Electric Smart Meters: Not a Smart Solution for Your Health?*, s.v. "thetruthaboutcancer.com electric smart meters," https://thetruthaboutcancer.com/electric-smart-meters/ (accessed 2019).
19	Quantum Spanner, *Nikola Tesla	The Father of Scalar Energy*, s.v. "www.quantumspanner.com tesla father of scalar energy," http://www.quantumspanner.com/tesla--father-of-scalar-energy.html (accessed 2019).
20	Spooky 2 Scalar, *History Of Scalar Energy*, s.v. "Spooky 2 Scalar history of scalar energy," https://www.spooky2scalar.com/history-of-scalar-energy/ (accessed 2019).
21	Lasota Energy, *What is Scalar energy?*, s.v. "Lasota Energy what is scalar energy," http://www.lasotaenergy.dk/wp-content/uploads/2014/11/Dokumentation-4.pdf (accessed 2019).
22	Lasota Energy, *What is Scalar energy?*, s.v. "Lasota Energy what is scalar energy," http://www.lasotaenergy.dk/wp-content/uploads/2014/11/Dokumentation-4.pdf (accessed 2019).
23	Scalar Energy Pendants, *Volcanic Rock Energy Pendant Will Boost Your Energy, Protects You From EMF Radiation & Much More*, s.v. "scalar energy pendants volcanic rock," https://www.scalarenergypendants.com/ (accessed 2019).
24	Lasota Energy, *What is Scalar energy?*, s.v. "Lasota Energy what is scalar energy," http://www.lasotaenergy.dk/wp-content/uploads/2014/11/Dokumentation-4.pdf (accessed 2019).
25	Frequency Energy 1 w/ the Universe, *Scalar Waves*, s.v. "Frequency Energy scalar waves," http://freqe1.com/the-scalar-factor/scalar-waves/ (accessed 2019).
26	Baseline of Health Foundation, *Scalar Energy, A Natural Alternative	Special Report*, s.v. "Baseline of Health Foundation scalar energy," https://jonbarron.org/article/energy-life (accessed 2017).
27	Baseline of Health Foundation, *Scalar Energy, A Natural Alternative	Special Report*, s.v. "Baseline of Health Foundation scalar energy," https://jonbarron.org/article/energy-life (accessed 2017).

Chapter 10

28	YouTube (video), iHealthTube (posted July 18, 2011), *Chemotherapy is a Waste of Money*, s.v. "Dr. Peter Glidden video Chemotherapy is a Waste of Money," https://www.youtube.com/watch?v=XdLyMhNdcSc (accessed 2017).
29	MDS Foundation (video), *Animation—Understanding Myelodysplastic Syndromes*, s.v. "what are primary and secondary MDS," http://www.youandmds.com/en-mds/view/m101-a01-understanding-myelodysplastic-syndromes-animation (accessed 2019).
30	MDS Foundation, *What is MDS?*, s.v. "what is MDS," https://www.mds-foundation.org/what-is-mds (accessed 2018).
31	MDS Foundation, *What is MDS?*, s.v. "what is MDS," https://www.mds-foundation.org/what-is-mds (accessed 2018).
32	MDS Foundation, *What is MDS?*, s.v. "what is MDS," https://www.mds-foundation.org/what-is-mds (accessed 2018).
33	Chemocare, Drug Information (menu tab), s.v. "Chemocare drug information," http://chemocare.com/ (accessed 2017).
34	American Association for Cancer Research, AACR Publications, *A History of Cancer Chemotherapy*, s.v. "A History of Cancer Chemotherapy 1943," https://cancerres.aacrjournals.org/content/68/21/8643 (accessed 2019).
35	*Wikipedia, Cyclophosphamide*, s.v. "cyclophosphamide 1959," https://en.wikipedia.org/wiki/Cyclophosphamide (accessed 2019).
36	*Wikipedia, Carboplatin*, s.v. "carboplatin 1972," https://en.wikipedia.org/wiki/Carboplatin (accessed 2019).
37	*Wikipedia, Etoposide*, s.v. "etoposide 1983," https://en.wikipedia.org/wiki/Etoposide (accessed 2019).
38	*Wikipedia, Paclitaxel*, s.v. "paclitaxel 1993," https://en.wikipedia.org/wiki/Paclitaxel (accessed 2019).
39	The Daily Beast, *Are We Wasting Billions Seeking a Cure for Cancer?*, s.v. "Are We Wasting Billions Seeking a Cure for Cancer," https://www.thedailybeast.com/are-we-wasting-billions-seeking-a-cure-for-cancer (accessed 2019).
40	NIH (National Institutes of Health), National Cancer Institute, *DCTD Division of Cancer Treatment & Diagnosis*, s.v. "DCTD Division of Cancer Treatment &

	Diagnosis pay for drug studies," https://dctd.cancer.gov/default.htm (accessed 2017).
41	BBC News, *Pharmaceutical industry gets high on fat profits*, s.v. "BBC News Pharmaceutical industry gets high on fat profits," https://www.bbc.com/news/business-28212223 (accessed 2019).
42	Bloomberg Businessweek, *Big Pharma Faces the Curse of the Billion-Dollar Blockbuster*, s.v. "Big Pharma Faces the Curse of the Billion-Dollar Blockbuster," https://www.bloomberg.com/news/articles/2019-01-11/big-pharma-faces-the-curse-of-the-billion-dollar-blockbuster (accessed 2019).
43	The Economist, *Clinical trials: Spilling the beans, Failure to publish the results of all clinical trials is skewing medical science*, s.v. "The Economist spilling the beans," https://www.economist.com/science-and-technology/2015/07/25/spilling-the-beans (accessed 2019).

Chapter 11

44	Cancer.Net, *What is a Bone Marrow Transplant (Stem Cell Transplant)?*, s.v. "What is a Bone Marrow Transplant (Stem Cell Transplant)," https://www.cancer.net/navigating-cancer-care/how-cancer-treated/bone-marrowstem-cell-transplantation/what-stem-cell-transplant-bone-marrow-transplant (accessed 2018).
45	Bishop Hussey, Diane, s.v. "Diane Bishop Hussey Crusade Against Cancers," https://www.dianebishophussey.com.
46	Dana-Farber Cancer Institute, *What happens during the stem cell transplant process?*, s.v. "what happens during the stem cell transplant process," https://www.dana-farber.org/health-library/articles/what-happens-during-the-stem-cell-transplant-process-/ (accessed 2019).
47	YouTube (video), Burzynski Movie (posted November 4, 2012), *Burzynski: Cancer Is Serious Business	Full Documentary	CANCER CURE*, s.v. "Burzynski: Cancer Is Serious Business documentary video," https://www.youtube.com/watch?v=rBUGVkmmwbk (accessed 2017).

Chapter 12

50	American Cancer Society, *What Is Acute Myeloid Leukemia (AML)?*, s.v. "what is acute myeloid leukemia," https://www.cancer.org/cancer/acute-myeloid-leukemia/about/what-is-aml.html (accessed 2017).
51	Cleveland Clinic Center for Continuing Education, *Hematology, Oncology, and Pulmonary Nodules*, s.v. "what does a spiculated edge indicate," http://www.clevelandclinicmeded.com/medicalpubs/diseasemanagement/hematology-oncology/pulmonary-nodules/ (accessed 2017).

Chapter 13

52	Budwig Center - A Natural Integrative Treatment Cancer Clinic, *Budwig Center Wellness Cancer Guide* (2011 guide may not available online), s.v. "Budwig Guide," http://www.budwigcenter.com/wp-content/uploads/2016/10/Johanna-Budwig-Guide-natural-therapies.pdf.
53	The Truth About Cancer, *Do You Have Low Iodine? The Link Between Iodine Deficiency & Cancer*, s.v. "link between iodine deficiency and cancer," https://thetruthaboutcancer.com/low-iodine-cancer/ (accessed 2019).
54	Cancer Fighting Strategies, *Oxygen and Cancer: Low Levels of Oxygen Can Breed Cancer*, s.v. "low oxygen and cancer," https://www.cancerfightingstrategies.com/oxygen-and-cancer.html (accessed 2019).
55	NIH (National Institutes of Health), National Cancer Institute, *The Genetics of Cancer*, s.v. "the genetics of cancer," https://www.cancer.gov/about-cancer/causes-prevention/genetics (accessed 2019). *(The Genetics of Cancer was originally published by the National Cancer Institute.)*
56	Showbiz CheatSheet, *15 Jobs That Put You at a Higher Risk of Cancer*, s.v. "jobs that put you at a higher risk of cancer," https://www.cheatsheet.com/money-career/jobs-put-higher-cancer-risk.html/ (accessed 2019).
57	WebMD, *Genes vs. Lifestyle: What Matters Most for Health?*, s.v. "Genes vs. Lifestyle: What Matters Most for Health," https://www.webmd.com/healthy-aging/features/genes-or-lifestyle (accessed 2019).
58	Cancer Tutor, *Step 2: What Causes Cancer?*, s.v. "CancerTutor What Causes Cancer," https://www.cancertutor.com/what_causes_cancer/ (accessed 2017).
59	MedicineNet, *Medical Definition of Apoptosis*, s.v. "medical definition of apoptosis," https://www.medicinenet.com/script/main/art.asp?articlekey=11287 (accessed 2018).

60	Glidden ND, Dr. Peter, s.v. "Dr. Peter Glidden ND," https://www.glidden.healthcare/ (accessed 2017).
61	Healthline, *Monk Fruit Sweetener: Good or Bad?*, s.v. "is monk fruit sweetener good or bad," https://www.healthline.com/nutrition/monk-fruit-sweetener (accessed 2019).
62	The Truth About Cancer (video), Jeffrey M. Smith (posted January 31, 2018), *Jeffrey Smith: Why Are GMOs Are Bad?*, s.v. "Jeffrey Smith: Why Are GMOs Are Bad? video," https://thetruthaboutcancer.com/why-are-gmos-bad-video/ (accessed 2019).
63	Non-GMO Project, *GMO Facts*, s.v. "Non-GMO Project GMO Facts," https://www.nongmoproject.org/gmo-facts/ (accessed 2019).
64	Newshub, *Frankenscience: Pig-human hybrids made in the lab*, s.v. "Frankenscience: Pig-human hybrids made in the lab," https://www.newshub.co.nz/home/world/2017/01/frankenscience-pig-human-hybrids-made-in-the-lab.html (accessed 2019).
65	Health24, *Your gut is the cornerstone of your immune system*, s.v. "Your gut is the cornerstone of your immune system," https://www.health24.com/Medical/Flu/Preventing-flu/your-gut-is-the-cornerstone-of-your-immune-system-20160318 (accessed 2019).
66	EcoWatch, *How Good Gut Health Can Boost Your Immune System*, s.v. "Dr. Mark Hyman How Good Gut Health Can Boost Your Immune System," https://www.ecowatch.com/how-good-gut-health-can-boost-your-immune-system-1882013643.html (accessed 2019).
67	NIH (National Institutes of Health), National Cancer Institute, *Radiation Therapy to Treat Cancer*, s.v. "Radiation Therapy to Treat Cancer," https://www.cancer.gov/about-cancer/treatment/types/radiation-therapy (accessed 2019).
68	NCBI (National Center for Biotechnology Information), US National Library of Medicine, National Institute of Health, *DNA Damage and Breast Cancer*, s.v. "DNA Damage and Breast Cancer," https://www.ncbi.nlm.nih.gov/pmc/articles/PMC3168783/ (accessed 2019).
69	NIH (National Institutes of Health), U.S. National Library of Medicine, ClinicalTrials.gov, *HBOT Late Radiation Tissue Injury*, s.v. "HBOT Late Radiation Tissue Injury," https://clinicaltrials.gov/ct2/show/NCT02425215 (accessed 2019).

70	Verywell Health, *Long-Term Side Effects of Radiation Therapy*, s.v. "Long-Term Side Effects of Radiation Therapy," https://www.verywellhealth.com/long-term-side-effects-of-radiation-therapy-2249293 (accessed 2019).
71	The Cancer Exchange, *Danger! Danger! Toxic Spill*, s.v. "The Cancer Exchange Danger! Danger! Toxic Spill," https://thecancerexchange.com/chemospill/ (accessed 2017).
72	NIH (National Institutes of Health), National Cancer Institute, SEER Training Modules, *Possible Side Effects*, s.v. "cancer side effects die-off of cells," https://training.seer.cancer.gov/treatment/chemotherapy/sideeffects.html (accessed 2017).
73	Mayo Clinic, *Cancer*, s.v. "cancer causes, gene mutations," https://www.mayoclinic.org/diseases-conditions/cancer/symptoms-cause/syc-20370588 (accessed 2017).
74	Cancer Research UK, *Genes, DNA and cancer*, s.v. "Genes, DNA and cancer," https://www.cancerresearchuk.org/about-cancer/what-is-cancer/genes-dna-and-cancer (accessed 2019).

Chapter 14

75	Budwig Center - A Natural Integrative Treatment Cancer Clinic, *Budwig Center Wellness Cancer Guide* (2011 guide may not available online), s.v. "Budwig Guide," http://www.budwigcenter.com/wp-content/uploads/2016/10/Johanna-Budwig-Guide-natural-therapies.pdf.
76	Budwig Center - A Natural Integrative Treatment Cancer Clinic, *Did Dr. Budwig Add Milk to The Flaxseed Oil and Cottage Cheese Recipe?*, s.v. "Did Dr. Budwig Add Milk to The Flaxseed Oil and Cottage Cheese Recipe," https://budwigcenter.com/dr-budwig-milk-flaxsees-oil-cottage-cheese-recipe (accessed 2019).
77	Budwig Center - A Natural Integrative Treatment Cancer Clinic, *Budwig Center Wellness Cancer Guide* (2011 guide may not available online), s.v. "Budwig Guide," http://www.budwigcenter.com/wp-content/uploads/2016/10/Johanna-Budwig-Guide-natural-therapies.pdf.
78	NaturalNews, *CT scans used to monitor success of cancer treatments cause more cancer, study finds*, s.v. "can CT scans cause cancer," https://www.naturalnews.com/032120_CT_scans_cancer.html (accessed 2019).

| 79 | American Cancer Society, *Do x-rays and gamma rays cause cancer?*, s.v. "do x-rays cause cancer," https://www.cancer.org/cancer/cancer-causes/radiation-exposure/x-rays-gamma-rays/do-xrays-and-gamma-rays-cause-cancer.html (accessed 2017). |

Chapter 16

| 81 | Budwig Center - A Natural Integrative Treatment Cancer Clinic, *Budwig Center Wellness Cancer Guide* (2011 guide may not be available online), s.v. "Budwig Guide raw chocolate fudge recipe," http://gbccct.org/wp-content/uploads/2019/04/A-BUDWIG-GUIDE-July-2015.pdf. |
| 82 | Medscape, *Guidelines Define Hemoglobin Levels for Transfusion*, s.v. "hemoglobin levels for transfusion," http://www.medscape.com/viewarticle/760919 (accessed 2017). |

Chapter 17

83	BeatCancer.org, *5 Reasons Cancer Cells and Sugar Are Best Friends*, s.v. "5 Reasons Cancer Cells and Sugar Are Best Friends," https://beatcancer.org/blog-posts/5-reasons-cancer-and-sugar-are-best-friends/ (accessed 2019).
84	YouTube (video), Burzynski Movie (posted November 4, 2012), *Burzynski: Cancer Is Serious Business	Full Documentary	CANCER CURE*, s.v. "Burzynski: Cancer Is Serious Business documentary video," https://www.youtube.com/watch?v=rBUGVkmmwbk (accessed 2017).
85	WorldHealth.Net, *Red Alert: FDA Set to Ban Your Supplements*, s.v. "RED ALERT: FDA Set to Ban Your Supplements," https://worldhealth.net/forum/topic/462/ (accessed 2017).

Chapter 18

| 86 | *Wikipedia, Hippocratic Oath*, s.v. "complete wording of Hippocratic Oath," https://en.wikipedia.org/wiki/Hippocratic_Oath (accessed 2018). |

Chapter 19

| 87 | Cancer Tutor, *Jim Kelmun Protocol Supplemental*, s.v. "Jim Kelmun Protocol Supplemental," |

	https://www.cancertutor.com/kelmun/ (accessed 2017).

Chapter 20

89	TheDashPoem.com (poem), Ellis, Linda, *The Dash*, https://thedashpoem.com/ (accessed 2017). (*The Dash*, by Linda Ellis, Copyright © Inspire Kindness, 1996, thedashpoem.com)
91	Poets.org (poem), Gibran, Kahlil, *On Death*, s.v. "Kahlil Gibran poem on death," https://poets.org/poem/death (accessed 2017).

Chapter 22

93	World Affairs, *How Rockefeller Founded Modern Medicine and Killed Natural Cures*, s.v. "How Rockefeller Founded Modern Medicine and Killed Natural Cures," https://worldaffairs.blog/2015/10/20/how-rockefeller-founded-modern-medicine-and-killed-natural-cures/ (accessed 2018).
94	Natural Society, *John D. Rockefeller's American Cancer Society Never Meant to 'CURE' Cancer*, s.v. "John D. Rockefeller's American Cancer Society Never Meant to 'CURE' Cancer," http://naturalsociety.com/john-d-rockefeller-founded-american-cancer-society-1913-never-meant-cure-cancer/ (accessed 2018).
95	Healing Cancer Naturally, *The Hoxsey Legend*, s.v. "Healing Cancer Naturally, The John and Harry Hoxsey Legend," www.healingcancernaturally.com/medical-history.html (accessed 2018).
96	The Truth About Cancer, *The Suppression of a Natural Cancer Cure*, s.v. "The Truth About Cancer Ty Bollinger, The Suppression of a Natural Cancer Cure," https://thetruthaboutcancer.com/howard-hoxsey-natural-cancer-cures/ (accessed 2018).
97	WantToKnow.info, *Royal Rife Case Shows Discovering a Cure for Cancer Can Be Dangerous to Your Health*, s.v. "Royal Rife Case Shows Discovering a Cure for Cancer Can Be Dangerous to Your Health," www.wanttoknow.info/cancercuresroyalrife (accessed 2017).
98	Health Nut News, *Dr. Max Gerson . . . A cure that cost his life*, s.v. "Health Nut News, Dr. Max Gerson . . . A cure that cost his life," https://www.healthnutnews.com/dr-max-gerson-cure-cost-life/ (accessed 2018).

99	Health Nut News, *Dr. Max Gerson . . . A cure that cost his life*, s.v. "Health Nut News, Dr. Max Gerson . . . A cure that cost his life," https://www.healthnutnews.com/dr-max-gerson-cure-cost-life/ (accessed 2018).
100	Health Nut News, *Unintended Holistic Doctor Death Series: Over 90 Dead*, s.v. "Unintended Holistic Doctor Death Series: Over 90 Dead," https://www.healthnutnews.com/recap-on-my-unintended-series-the-holistic-doctor-deaths/ (accessed 2018).
101	CBS News, *Merck Created Hit List to Destroy Neutralize or Discredit Dissenting Doctors*, s.v. "Merck Created Hit List," https://www.cbsnews.com/news/merck-created-hit-list-to-destroy-neutralize-or-discredit-dissenting-doctors/ (accessed 2019).
102	MedPage Today, *It's Official! Curing Patients Is Bad for Business*, s.v. "Curing Patients Is Bad for Business," https://www.medpagetoday.com/blogs/revolutionandrevelation/72407 (accessed 2019).
103	Chicago Tribune, *Chicago water: In public water reports, city silent over sex hormones and painkillers found in treated drinking water*, s.v. "sex hormones and painkillers Chicago water," https://www.chicagotribune.com/lifestyles/health/chi-water-testing-14-jul14-story.html (accessed 2017).
104	Chicago Monitor, *Danger of Pharmaceuticals in Chicago's Water Supply*, s.v. "Pharmaceuticals in Chicago's Water Supply," http://chicagomonitor.com/2016/06/danger-of-pharmaceuticals-in-chicagos-water-supply/ (accessed 2019).
105	Pharma-Cycle, *Environmental impact of cytotoxic drugs that pass through patients*, s.v. "Environmental impact of cytotoxic drugs Pharma-Cycle," http://www.pharma-cycle.com/environdangers.html (accessed 2019).
106	Pharma-Cycle, *Environmental impact of cytotoxic drugs that pass through patients*, s.v. "Environmental impact of cytotoxic drugs Pharma-Cycle," http://www.pharma-cycle.com/environdangers.html (accessed 2019).
107	Pharma-Cycle, *Environmental impact of cytotoxic drugs that pass through patients*, s.v. "Environmental impact of cytotoxic drugs Pharma-Cycle," http://www.pharma-cycle.com/environdangers.html (accessed 2019).

108	ecoRI, *Chemo Drugs Pose Serious Public Health Risks*, s.v. "Chemo Drugs Pose Serious Public Health Risks," https://www.ecori.org/public-safety/2012/11/19/chemo-drugs-pose-serious-public-health-risks.html (accessed 2019).
109	Mullowney, Jim, s.v. "Jim Mullowney Pharma-Cycle," http://www.pharma-cycle.com.
110	Pharma-Cycle, *Environmental impact of cytotoxic drugs that pass through patients*, s.v. "Environmental impact of cytotoxic drugs Pharma-Cycle," http://www.pharma-cycle.com/environdangers.html (accessed 2019).
111	YouTube (video), TEDx Talks (posted January 23, 2017), *We Put a Man on the Moon | Jim Mullowney | TEDxNewport*, s.v. "We Put a Man on the Moon Jim Mullowney video," https://www.youtube.com/watch?v=zX6OsvzZdOw&t=135s (accessed 2019).
112	YouTube (video), Cytotoxic Safety Counsel (posted April 30, 2015), *FULL TESTIMONY - RI Senate Bill S0169 Hearing 4 11 15*, s.v. "FULL TESTIMONY - RI Senate Bill S0169 Hearing 4 11 15," https://www.youtube.com/watch?v=Nq65Nh1WMj0&t=335s (accessed 2019).
113	NIH (National Institutes of Health), National Cancer Institute, *The Genetics of Cancer*, s.v. "The Genetics of Cancer," https://www.cancer.gov/about-cancer/causes-prevention/genetics (accessed 2019). *(The Genetics of Cancer was originally published by the National Cancer Institute.)*
114	YouTube (video), Cytotoxic Safety Counsel (posted April 30, 2015), *FULL TESTIMONY - RI Senate Bill S0169 Hearing 4 11 15*, s.v. "FULL TESTIMONY - RI Senate Bill S0169 Hearing 4 11 15," https://www.youtube.com/watch?v=Nq65Nh1WMj0&t=335s (accessed 2019).

Chapter 23

115	Petersen, Melody. *Our Daily Meds: How the Pharmaceutical Companies Transformed Themselves into Slick Marketing Machines and Hooked the Nation on Prescription Drugs*, First Edition. New York: Picador, 2009.
116	MedicineNet, *Graft Versus Host Disease*, s.v. "graft versus host disease," https://www.medicinenet.com/graft_versus_host_disease_gvhd/article.htm#what_are_graft-versus-host_disease_symptoms_and_signs_what_are_the_types_of_gvhd (accessed 2018).

117	Mayo Clinic, *Bone Marrow Transplant*, s.v. "Mayo Clinic bone marrow transplant overview," https://www.mayoclinic.org/tests-procedures/bone-marrow-transplant/about/pac-20384854 (accessed 2018).
118	YouTube (video), Bruce Sol Lee, *Patch Adams Complete Speech* (posted March 24, 2015), s.v. "Patch Adams Complete Speech video," https://www.youtube.com/watch?v=KDEjgOFOLho (accessed 2019).
119	YouTube (video), joel10000a, *Ian McCormack - an Atheist - Dead on Morgue Slab - Goes to Hell, then to Heaven and Back!!* (posted March 2, 2011), s.v. "Ian McCormack dead on a slab video," https://www.youtube.com/watch?v=59mRZ1Vj8ZU (accessed 2017).
120	iHealthTube (video), *10 Questions You Must Ask Your Doctor Before Starting Cancer Treatments!*, s.v. "10 Questions You Must Ask Your Doctor Before Starting Cancer Treatments iHealthTube," https://www.ihealthtube.com/video/10-questions-you-must-ask-your-doctor-starting-cancer-treatments (accessed 2018).
121	Bishop Hussey, Diane, s.v. "Diane Bishop Hussey Crusade Against Cancers," https://www.dianebishophussey.com.

About the Author

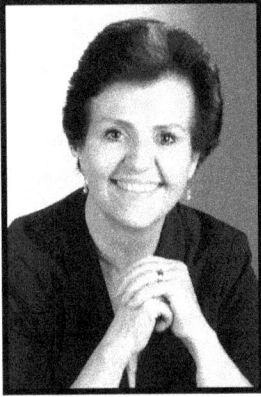

Author and speaker Diane Bishop Hussey is on a mission to raise awareness about cancer and bring the truth to light.

Diane has been involved with natural health since 2009. She received the designation of Certified Natural Health Counselor (CNHC) in 2011 and Registered Natural Health Practitioner (RNHP) in 2012. In 2016 Diane spoke at the International Association of Natural Health Practitioners Conference.

In addition, she is an ordained chaplain with an associate's degree in ministry.

Diane lives in Illinois near her elderly parents, while her three children are scattered around the country. She is positive and upbeat, telling friends and strangers alike, "Choose your attitude, and make it a good one!"

For more information about working with Diane as a natural health counselor, visit www.DianeBishopHussey.com.

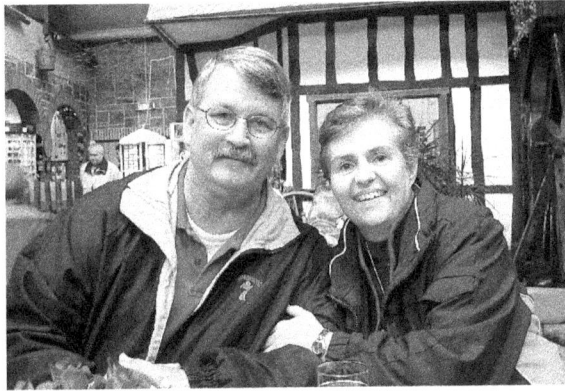

www.ingramcontent.com/pod-product-compliance
Lightning Source LLC
Chambersburg PA
CBHW080325270326
41927CB00014B/3101